DANGER TO SELF

DANGER TO SELF

ON THE FRONT LINE
WITH AN ER PSYCHIATRIST

PAUL R. LINDE, MD

UNIVERSITY OF CALIFORNIA PRESS

BERKELEY LOS ANGELES LONDON

University of California Press, one of the most distinguished university presses in the United States, enriches lives around the
world by advancing scholarship in the humanities, social sciences,
and natural sciences. Its activities are supported by the UC Press
Foundation and by philanthropic contributions from individuals
and institutions. For more information, visit www.ucpress.edu.

University of California Press
Berkeley and Los Angeles, California

University of California Press, Ltd.
London, England

Library of Congress Cataloging-in-Publication Data
Linde, Paul R.
    Danger to self : on the front line with an ER psychiatrist / Paul R.
Linde.
        p.   cm.
    Includes bibliographical references.
    ISBN 978-0-520-24984-4 (cloth : alk. paper)
    1. Psychiatric emergencies—Popular works.   I. Title.
    [DNLM: 1. Emergency Services, Psychiatric—Personal
Narratives.   2. Crisis Intervention—Personal Narratives.
3. Mental Disorders—diagnosis—Personal Narratives.
4. Mental Disorders—therapy—Personal Narratives.   5. Mentally
Ill Persons—psychology—Personal Narratives.   6. Physician's
Role—Personal Narratives.   WM 401 L7427d 2010]
    RC480.6.L557   2010
    616.89'025—dc22   2009006144

Manufactured in the United States of America

19 18 17 16 15 14 13 12 11 10
10 9 8 7 6 5 4 3 2 1

This book is printed on Cascades Enviro 100, a 100% post con-
sumer waste, recycled, de-inked fiber. FSC recycled certified and
processed chlorine free. It is acid free, Ecologo certified, and manufactured by BioGas energy.

For my boys, Jacob and Sam

True happiness, we are told, consists in getting out of one's self; but the point is not only to get out—you must stay out; and to stay out you must have some absorbing errand.

Henry James, *Roderick Hudson,* 1875

CONTENTS

ACKNOWLEDGMENTS

I especially thank the gracious writers, readers, and editors who vetted various drafts of the manuscript and spent precious hours helping me to conceptualize, contextualize, and process not only a whole lot of technical information but also emotionally laden material, of which there was no shortage.

Much credit is due to my colleagues in the Sanchez Writers Grotto, especially its mastermind, Doug Wilkins, and writers extraordinaire Kemble Scott, Shana Mahaffey, Diane Weipert, Michael Chorost, Raj Patel, Melodie Bowsher, Alison Bing, Rob Tocalino, Sean Beaudoin, Michelle Gagnon, Ammi Keller, Bernice Yeung, Eric Tipler, and Joshua Citrak.

Other important readers and motivational figures include Paul Cohen, Audrey Ferber, David Brendel, Ellyn Saks, Tanya Luhrmann, Frank Huyler, Adam Bluestein, Ian Wheeler-Nicholson, Vikram Patel, Gauri Divan, Katherine Straznickas, Jeb Berkeley, and Paul Jones. Jane Dystel and Miriam Goderich gave me tremendous momentum while helping me deliver this project from the depths of my unconscious, and occasionally insane, mind.

Two colleagues, Bob Buckley and Isadore Talesnick, provided me with valuable interview material. Appreciation is also due to my physician colleagues—Drs. Buckley, John Rouse, Katrina Peters, John Harbison, John Herbert, Jo Ellen Brainin-Rodriguez, Laurie Richer, Rick Patel, Eric Woodard, David Elkin, Mark Schiller, Evan Garner, Elias Aboujaoude, Brad Novak, John Herbert, Jim Manning, Chad Peterson, Mark Leary, Francis Lu, James Dilley, and many others. Craig Van Dyke, Bob Okin, and Nicole Sawaya were also very helpful.

I also thank my multidisciplinary colleagues at San Francisco General Hospital—nurses, psych techs, social workers, support staff, students, interns, residents, and the all-time MVP of the place, Romeo Tagle—for making my time in psych emergency memorable and, when not gut-busting, gut-splitting.

My personal editor, Amy Bianco, was incredibly kind to help me sharpen my concepts, polish my language, and figure out the chapter order.

I very kindly thank my editor at the University of California Press, Naomi Schneider, who saw potential in a somewhat nebulously formulated book proposal. I'm glad she took a chance on me and had enough of that "vision thing" to help me get this thing done. I am also grateful to Laura Harger and Bonita Hurd for making the book clearer, cleaner, and more appealing.

In particular, I am indebted to my father, Lew Linde, and my now-deceased mother, Marcella Ruhr Linde, and my brothers and sisters, Ken, Kay, Rick, and Sara, back in Minnesota. Special gratitude goes to all my wonderful friends in San Francisco and elsewhere, my boys, Jacob and Sammy, and, of course, my wife, Laurie Schultz. Without her support, the ideas for this book would never have come to fruition. Thank you.

NOWHERE TO HIDE

A doctor, however, who would still interpret his own role mainly as
that of a technician would confess that he sees in his patient nothing
more than a machine, instead of seeing the human being behind the
disease!

Viktor Frankl, *Man's Search for Meaning*

I love my job when I'm not there. I'm a doctor in the psych
emergency room at San Francisco General Hospital (SFGH).
One reason I work there is that when I'm not there, I'm not
there. I have a decent shot at separating out my job's trauma and
drama from the rest of my life. But in my workplace, there's
nowhere to hide.

Our staff room, which provides a slight refuge, is dominated
by a huge table, dozens of mailboxes and forms along one wall,
a copier, a fax machine, shelves of books, a little sink (over which
hangs the requisite "Your mother doesn't work here" sign), a
microwave, a tiny fridge, an illicit toaster, food and drink rem-
nants, and the computer monitors on which we keep electronic
medical records. Up to fifteen administrators, staff members,
interns, residents, and students might be stuffed in this approximately ten-by-fourteen-foot place at any one time. The space is

not secured within a Plexiglas fish bowl, as are staff rooms in many psychiatric units, but instead is open to the patients, walled off only by a modest counter and half-door about four feet high. Patients do wander in from time to time, and at least two have been known to jump the wall in a single bound—one to sucker punch a nurse, the other to escape out of a slightly ajar first-story window. It's a twenty-four-seven, all-day-every-day place.

The SFGH Psychiatric Emergency Service (PES) is primarily an evaluation unit for patients involuntarily held for up to three days for a psychiatric assessment and a period of observation. More than half of our patients have been detained, under civil but not criminal code, and brought in by the police. California's Welfare and Institutions Code section 5150 provides the legal justification for a person to be involuntarily taken into custody for up to seventy-two hours to evaluate whether he or she is a danger to self, a danger to others, and/or gravely disabled because of a psychiatric illness.

Many patients feel, often justifiably, that they are treated as miscreants when their only "crime" is that of suffering symptoms of mental illness. As you can imagine, an individual confined on these grounds may be upset, to put it mildly, about being locked up against his or her will in the absence of criminal charges.

The front door to the place is locked—you need a key to get in and out, unless you get buzzed through a double set of doors separated by a sally port. It's not unlike a DMZ. Before entry, police officers check their guns, placing them in a small locker—similar to a bank safety deposit box—built into the wall outside the front door of psych emergency.

PES is licensed by the state to hold and observe a maximum of eighteen patients for up to twenty-four hours. In reality, from time to time we confine patients for two or three days, and our census sometimes jumps into the midtwenties. What else can we do with psychiatrically unstable patients who can't be safely returned to the community and who have nowhere else to go?

Patients brought into PES are already on edge, their emotions intensified and jangled. But raw feelings of the staff also come to the surface in a work environment complete with unbearable mounds of paperwork, unreasonable rules about county residency and benefits, and obstacles constructed by private insurance companies, which, it seems, spend more money denying care than they do providing care.

Sometimes all a doctor or nurse can do is respond to behavioral emergencies in the moment: head banging; temper tantrums with the menace of violence; the monolithic man who breaks through his heavy metal seclusion-room door; the woman who nearly bites her finger off; the delirious, febrile, HIV-positive man who cuts his wrist with a paper clip and spurts blood at the staff; the smearing of feces; the attempted hangings in the bathroom; the throwing of heavy plastic chairs.

"Treating psychiatric patients can be a nearly impossible task," writes T. M. Luhrmann in her landmark book *Of Two Minds: An Anthropologist Looks at American Psychiatry.* "Those who do so often collapse with foxhole hilarity around the stress."[1] True. But when I'm not collapsing, I'm revving up. The place *does* harbor, nay, encourage, a manic-depressive character. I bounce out of my chair from time to time, sometimes because I simply feel a need to move my body, but just as often because there is a medical or behavioral fire to put out. I occasionally situate myself in front of the nursing station—between the shift's charge nurse and the doors of our four seclusion rooms. I am one part bouncer, one part traffic cop, one part standup comedian, and one part maître d'. "Sedative, anyone?"

This psychiatric job requires a certain amount of physicality. I am on my feet a lot, trying to soothe the jangled nerves of the weary, the sick, and the stressed—the latter category often includes the staff. Working in PES can be compared to diving into the swirl of a cyclone and hanging on for dear life. You adjust to the velocity and spin enough to manage as many as four equally compelling tasks at the same time. It helps to arrive equipped with the unusual combination of a short attention span and an ability to concentrate deeply in the midst of pandemonium. Out of your mouth pours a telephone discussion with the medical ER's physician-in-charge regarding a dehydrated catatonic patient. Into one ear floods the story of a suicidal elderly man with terminal cancer and chronic pain. And in the background reverberate the screamed profanities of your newest patient and the rumbling, rattling cough of another one who may have tested positive for tuberculosis.

If you try to make sense of the place, you'll lose your mind. If you don't sweat the details, you can get a patient in trouble. If you do sweat the details, you'll run out of time.

I say I'm crazy in order to ward off actually becoming crazy. As a stress management technique, I sometimes say the same things over and over and over again, almost like Dustin Hoffman in *Rain Man*. It's a form of self-soothing. It's a defense. It's called regression in the service of the ego, which is a fancy way of saying, "I need to blow off a lot of steam along the way" to keep my mental and emotional engine from overheating or breaking down in the face of the chronic stress and unpredictability of psych emergency.

People can understand the tragedy of being in a car accident or getting cancer. The doctors who treat such patients, trauma surgeons and oncologists, can easily acquire the patina of heroism. I give those doctors their due. They do incredibly important work. But people don't consider psych emergency doctors in the same light. People do not want to think of the possibility of being felled by schizophrenia, bipolar disorder, or disabling depression. "Sure, those things happen to other people, in other families, but they do not happen to me or my family members."

In darker moments, doctors and nurses employed in psychiatric emergency have occasionally maligned our own work as meatball psychiatry or, with apologies to my animal-doctor colleagues, veterinary psychiatry. Yet our work is anything but. We know the stakes are high for our patients, and that they are undoubtedly having one of the worst days of their lives. We simply use multiple psychological defenses to get through the shift. Those pejorative shorthand descriptions of the task at hand, part of medicine's long-standing tradition of gallows humor, should be seen for what they truly are—maladaptive defenses of the psyche against the intensity and pathos of the problems we face every day.

In fact, our work is deeply rooted in respect for the patient. Most of us want to help people who often have been left behind and forgotten by society. We are guides to a bewildering healthcare system in which acronyms predominate and the rules change often. We all play a shell game of sorts with services that are here today but gone tomorrow. The system of public mental health care in the United States has been maimed and is dying slowly—death by a thousand cuts.

Shame, secrecy, and stigma surround psychiatric illness and even the people associated with it—those crazy psychiatrists. Better to set mental illness to the side, keep it at a distance. It might be catching. I often hear some variation of this: "You work where? How can you stand it?" Many civilians—the rubberneckers and disaster junkies—express a morbid fascination with the subject: "Wow, you must see some really crazy shit, huh? Tell me the craziest thing you ever saw!" And I usually answer, "Well, that's a tough one" or "I don't know, there's so many" or "Geez, I hate to think about my work when I'm not there."

Upon hearing where I work, a taxi driver tells me point-blank, "Wow. Either you're a generous person or a glutton for punishment."

"Well, I'm a little bit of both, I'm afraid."

In contrast, nonpsychiatric health professionals usually say things like "I could never do that. Thank God you guys are there." Society as a whole would much prefer not knowing what happens behind the closed doors of psychiatric emergency. It could happen to you. There but for the grace of God go you, your partner, child, sibling, parent, uncle, aunt, grandparent, cousin. Severe psychiatric illness can happen to anyone. Maybe that's why people would rather shield their eyes from the glow of this reality.

On the surface, this book demonstrates the nature of my work as a psychiatrist in a wide variety of settings, but mostly in the psychiatric emergency room at SFGH. It shows the kind of tasks given to me, what I do, how I talk to patients, how I think, and how I make decisions in situations that can best be described as knotty, enigmatic, and almost never routine. When all is said and done, society is paying me to exercise my best professional judgment in trying to solve seemingly insoluble problems. My decisions are made in a financially deprived and pressurized environment, often with incomplete data, and the tasks are rife with ethical dilemmas. Though I am, of course, obliged to be an able and compassionate colleague, supervisor, teacher, and practitioner, I mostly get paid to make good decisions as a proxy for society as a whole.

I provide a skill set, experience, and a willingness that few others can give to the work. It's not a popular place of employment for most psychiatrists, but instead is a way station on the road to more illustrious careers. Yet, even though the outcomes of my work are qualitative, vague, and uncertain, I find my job a satisfying one on a moment-to-moment basis as I do my best to help society's most disenfranchised and hopeless. The task is a grave but wonderful challenge.

As you read this book, you will no doubt see the setting of psych emergency for what it can be: loud, chaotic, smelly, messy, and dangerous, among other things. And you will sense the tension inherent in the work. But you will also see the redeeming essence of the work: the moment-to-moment relationship between doctor and patient.

What kind of doctor becomes an emergency psychiatrist? A psychiatrist friend of mine once said, "You guys who work in PES are good at chatting people up—kind of like a bartender. It's your job to make people feel comfortable right away." Of course, I'm serving up rapid-onset tranquilizers instead of martinis, but his comparison is a valid one.

My mentor in the psych ER, Dr. Bob Buckley, differentiates emergency psychiatrists from other psychiatrists in this way: "I think a lot of psychiatrists are reflective, maybe a little obsessive. There's not that many of us who are cowboys. You've got to have a little bit of cowboy in you to survive for very long in psych emergency. You've got to have, for a psychiatrist, a kind of a reckless attitude." In other words, you've got to be a little bit out there, unafraid to go out on a limb from time to time.

The surgeon-author Richard Selzer writes, "If all Medicine be considered a religion, why, then, the psychiatrist is the cloistered nun, a contemplative whose pale hands are unused save for the telling of beads. The surgeon is burly, brawling Friar Tuck, out in the world, taking up his full share of space, and always at some risk of exposing rather too much of his free-swinging beef from beneath his habit."[2] I've always behaved much more like the meaty, beaty, big, and bouncy surgeon than the navel-gazing psychiatrist. This is partly the result of a body habitus that's ranged from 200 to 260 pounds on a five-foot-eleven-inch frame during my career as a psychiatrist. It's a little hard to hide an ascetic persona in that frame.

While the book is part memoir, part primer, and part commentary, what I am most interested in is documenting my experiences and those of my patients. I search for verisimilitude; I aim to capture the essence of the work. But in doing this I am, of course, required to strike a delicate balance between getting the real story out and protecting the confidentiality of patients, without sacrificing the essential truths that I explore. The patient stories in each chapter are closely based on actual events and circumstances. In other words, they really happened. However, to protect the privacy and confidentiality of patients who've been evaluated and treated in the psych emergency setting, identifying characteristics such as age, gender, ethnicity,

housing situation, marital status, occupation, and religious preference were often changed to obscure the actual identity of individual patients. The names of some of the nurses were changed
to protect their privacy.

The dialogue as presented here was not transcribed from
audio recordings. Taping patient interviews in the psych emergency setting (and in most psychiatric clinical environments) is
considered illegal, unethical, and a breach of confidentiality.
Because of this, the conversations presented here have been
reconstructed from memory. Every attempt has been made to
follow a credible line of inquiry between doctor and patient and
to capture the general tone of those interactions.

I wrote this book for the educated lay reader. It is a work of
commercial—dare I say literary?—nonfiction. It is in no way
intended to be a comprehensive perspective on emergency psychiatry. Though I provide citations to identify sources of quotes
and to support certain statistical facts, the book is not meant
to be a scholarly work. Topics such as civil commitment law,
malingering, violence, cognitive neurosciences, the nature of
consciousness, and suicide are areas of concentration suitable for
full-length academic books. These topics can be only superfi-
cially summarized, at best, within the confines of narrative-
driven chapters like the ones I offer here.

The first chapter in this book details my introduction to psych
emergency in 1992, my first day on the job as a fully trained
attending psychiatrist. The next three stories in this collection,
chapters 2 through 4, reach back in time, occurring between
1988 and 1992, during my internship and residency at the
University of California, San Francisco's School of Medicine.
The first narrative describes a hair-raising experience I had

while moonlighting at the county jail. The second illustrates my reaction to a potentially homicidal patient in my office. And the third chronicles my fledgling attempts at learning to become a psychotherapist.

The remaining chapters are organized as much by theme as they are by chronology. Chapters 5 through 7 not only give you a greater sense of the atmosphere and problems experienced in a place like psych emergency, but they also provide a context in which to understand the complex decisions and value judgments that acute care psychiatrists must make. These chapters touch on fundamental existential questions: What is the nature of freedom and autonomy? How does one protect an individual's civil liberties while also taking into account society's need for public safety and its responsibility to help those who are sick and less fortunate? Who "deserves" treatment? When is it morally justifiable to revoke a person's right to freedom, to autonomy? What are the historical and legal contexts in which these decisions are made? Can psychiatrists accurately predict a person's behavior? How aggressive should a psychiatrist be in making decisions and delivering treatment?

Chapters 8 and 9 document two common problems seen in psych emergency—methamphetamine abuse and the lingering effects of childhood trauma. The questions explored in these two chapters include: Why do people use drugs? What is the nature of suffering? How does one cope with demoralization in the face of overwhelming life problems? How does one find resilience and a sense of meaning to counterbalance such things?

The tenth chapter is an outlier. It occurs in a different setting—with me as a consultant to a liver transplant team in the medical-surgical part of a private hospital. Yet it more deeply explores the questions of who deserves treatment and how scarce resources get distributed.

In writing this book, I discovered that psych emergency has cast a sort of spell over me. It's the place I've worked the longest, by far. For many of the mental health professionals who work there, myself included, the attraction to the place and the work borders on the obsessive. It's just too boring to work anywhere else. Even after living and working as a psychiatrist in Zimbabwe for a year in the mid-1990s—an experience that formed the basis of my first book, *Of Spirits and Madness: An American Psychiatrist in Africa*—I made a beeline to my next job in psych emergency.[3] I've been there ever since. The place drew me all the way out of Africa—a subconscious clarion call. Working in such a place as psych emergency is not just compelling but actually addicting.

Yet working there is one thing; writing about it is another. Mine is considered an out-of-sight, out-of-mind job for a reason. There were many, many days when I sat down to write about my work in psych emergency and nothing came out. Or I had to literally force my fingers to move across the keys. On other days I was in the mood to vent, and what came out was splenetic, bilious, over-the-top, sanctimonious—in a word, unusable. However, these eruptions proved cathartic—a laxative for the psyche, so to speak—and much, much cheaper than becoming a perennial Woody Allen manacled to an analytic couch.

On the face of it, *Danger to Self* refers to the physical dangers for both patients and staff—self-injury, suicide attempts, assaults, illness. But for legal purposes, "danger to self" means a risk of suicide or other self-harm. On a deeper level, the title refers to the emotional danger—of absorbing toxic energy with no outlet—inherent in the work of a psychiatrist, particularly an emergency psychiatrist. Occupational hazards for the modern-day psychiatrist include anxiety, depression, alcoholism, addiction, and emotional withdrawal. The writing of this book manifested an enormous psychological defense—the creation of an Other to counterbalance my shadow self. A deeper consideration of the day-to-day suffering that I witness and try to alleviate has forced me to confront my actual feelings about my chosen career, which are highlighted by ambivalence. Am I really the informal, irreverent jokester that I sometimes like to consider myself? Well, yes and no. The clown is also a persona, a defense, created to soothe and bandage raw emotions that are stirred by the serial suffering and tragedies that confront me daily in psych emergency. Is it me? Or is it a defense? Can it be both?

This book is intended to humanize psychiatrists, other mental health professionals, patients, and their loved ones. It is okay for psychiatrists and other mental health professionals to be ourselves with patients. It is okay at times to laugh, to swear, to self-reveal, to cry with our patients—to emphasize our humanity. It does not mean transgressing boundaries. This stance does not categorically detract from some idealized notion of what it means to be a professional. Detachment, woodenness, adherence to diagnostic checklists, therapeutic neutrality, and undue formality on the part of a psychiatrist all do much harm to a patient in the context of a clinical interaction that might otherwise offer a wonderful opportunity for healing.

I don't love my job. I don't hate my job. I am *not* my job when I am not there. I *am* my job when I am there. And therein the danger lies.

ONE

THE ER DOC

Who's Calling the Shots?

The activist psychiatrist R. D. Laing has this to say about the potentially coercive power invested in psychiatrists by society: "We should not blame psychiatrists because we give them such depth of power, especially when, to be exercised as expected, it *must* be exercised *routinely*."[1]

I guess we shouldn't blame psychiatric nurses, either. When I first started working as an attending psychiatrist at PES, I discovered that my most complicated workplace relationships were with many of the experienced nurses who worked there. They were the power players, and my education began even before I had worked a shift.

Throughout this book, it may seem as if psychiatric nurses and emergency psychiatrists are mentioned interchangeably. And that is no coincidence. In the psychiatric emergency setting, nurses and doctors work very closely, side by side, with each other. There is an egalitarian feel to the place. While it is the physician who has the final say and ultimate responsibility from a practical and a medicolegal perspective, it is a foolish emergency psychiatrist who does not collaborate with his or her knowledgeable and experienced psychiatric nurse colleagues in making clinical decisions.

I had my reasons for choosing to work in psych emergency—some of them logical, others psychological, and many still to be discovered. My first paying gig was low-stress—a doctors' staff meeting convened by PES's medical director. Though he had hired me, the medical director would never be my role model. The son of a diplomat, he carried himself stiffly, a jacket-and-tie kind of guy, the product of boarding schools. He did not manifest the roll-up-your-sleeves style that I imagined an effective emergency psychiatrist should possess.

. . .

My first night at work is an unseasonably warm evening in the summer of 1992. The customary layer of fog has not yet descended on the city. The psych emergency room is stuffy, the ventilation poor, the ceiling's air vents clogged with lint and dust. A faint whiff of fresh feces and old urine, ineffectively masked by a cloying cinnamon-scented spray, hangs about the place. It is then that I understand why state hospital psychiatrists smoke cigarettes on the job—to cut the stench. Though I had worked there for a week as a fourth-year resident just a few months earlier, this is my initial performance as an authority figure in psych emergency. At this point, I haven't worked a shift yet. I had just returned, lean and refreshed, from a month's holiday spent traveling with my wife in a 1984 Volkswagen camper van through the Pacific Northwest and the Rockies. I had enjoyed an invigorating taste of freedom on this trip, and now I was beginning my career on a lockdown. Though I was getting paid for my time and had chosen this vocational path, I was still working in a place for which a key was required to get out.

Uncharacteristically, I arrive about ten minutes early. Two nurses, a man and a woman, sit behind the triage desk, a crescent-shaped structure about four feet high and twelve feet long facing four seclusion rooms, each with a heavy metal locking door, and each containing a steel bed equipped with four leather belt restraints (these days the belts are made of washable polyester and Velcro), one per extremity. The lights are dimmed.

To the right of the desk is the triage area, accessible by passage through double locked doors. This is where the police and paramedics enter to bring in patients from the streets. To the left is the sprawling dayroom, really a twenty-four-seven room, in which patients sit and sleep on pull-out chairs. Behind the desk, separated by a wall with two doors, is the cramped staff room. Sitting at the desk, the two nurses look like commanders of a starship, which in fact they are, as many of the ward's denizens are in some sort of orbit, psychiatric or otherwise. Christina, the shift's charge nurse, invites me over for a chat and a chocolate-frosted doughnut, which I enthusiastically accept. I sit down and begin eating. "Well, Paul," she says, "what do you think of this *cray-zee* place?"

"I like it here," I say, dropping crumbs on my shirt. "I like the chaos." I already knew Christina from my weeklong rotation. She had worked there since the old days, starting in the late 1970s or early 1980s. It takes me only a few minutes to surmise that she has a knack for getting her way, does not suffer fools gladly, and is not to be trifled with.

"That's good," says the man sitting beside her, the shift's triage nurse, "because I'm sure you'll soon find out that the staff is near-lee as *cray-zee* as the patients." Bo, short for Beauregard, son of the South, giggles and sniffs twice before grooming his salt-and-pepper beard and adjusting his glasses in what seems like a single motion. "But I'm sure *you* can handle it."

"Oh, yeah," I say.

Just then the medical director walks by. I'm not sure if it's my imagination, but I think the director, normally flat and imperturbable, rolls his eyes and exhales ever so slightly when he sees me sitting next to the two nurses behind the desk. "Paul, the meeting starts in three minutes, so please join us," he says.

"Sure," I say, continuing to sit there. Once he is out of range, Christina turns to me and asks softly, "What do you think of *that* one?"

"Well, uh," I say, pausing, trying to think of something tactful.

"He's clueless," she says, not missing a beat. "A deforester. He's only good at creating new paperwork. He doesn't know a thing about what really goes on around here."

"Oh, *that* one," Bo says in a high-pitched Southern accent. "What a waste of training. If he'd just leave us alone, we'd be okay."

"Yeah, our last medical director was great," adds Christina. "He really knew his stuff. The patients loved him. But, Paul," she says, leaning closer, her voice dropping to a whisper, "*they* killed him off because he always took our side."

"Who are *they*?" I ask.

"*They* . . . are the administration," she says conspiratorially. "Especially the nursing leadership. *They* need to be in charge. Even though they don't know shit about what we do or what goes on down here." I had arrived during an era in which employee-management relationships in health care seemed

particularly precarious. The animosity ran both ways and con
tributed to the rising level of tension already inherent in a place
like psych emergency.

"Well," says Bo, "our last medical director also left us because
his wife was expecting and he could double his salary in
Wisconsin. But they did kill him off."

I nod. "I see."

Suddenly, a rather large, unkempt man, a scowl on his face,
stumbles out of one of the four seclusion rooms and ambles to
the desk.

"What do you want, George?" asks Christina.

"I need to take a piss."

"Get back in that room, or we'll have to tie your ass up and
give you a shot."

"But I need to go real bad."

"Get back in there. I'll bring you a urinal."

"I want to pee in a fuckin' toilet, not a fuckin' bottle."

"Get back in there, George. Now."

"Fuck you, you slanty-eyed bitch," he says as he comes half-
lurching, half-lunging toward the desk.

"Staff!" yell the nurses.

"For that," Bo says, "he's going into points." The shorthand
points is emergency room slang for the four points at which a
patient's extremities are attached via restraints to a bed bolted to
the floor of a seclusion room. I'm not sure, when Bo says "that,"
whether he's referring to the menacing stance or the racially
charged barb or the whole package.

Since I am not officially on duty and am new to the place and
generally inexperienced, I step back. Three staff members rush
to the scene and grab George by the hands and around the waist

and escort him roughly to his seclusion room, where he lies down on the bed without a struggle. "Do we need to call IP?" asks one. At the time, the hospital was staffed by bona fide San Francisco institutional police officers, whose station was next door. We called them often.

"Nah," says Christina as she deftly encircles one of George's wrists with the belt loop of a leather restraint. All four of George's extremities are now strapped by restraints. Seemingly accustomed to this routine, George lies passively, his body supine on a clean white sheet.

"George, why did you have to go and do this?" asks a psych tech. "You're gonna get a shot now, too."

"Yeah, but I'm allergic to Haldol."

"Sure, George, sure."

A nameless, faceless doctor wrote the order for restraints and Haldol. Or maybe he just signed an order that the nurse had written herself on an order sheet. That was standard operating procedure in those days. Sitting in the staff room would be some MD who was happy to sign whatever order was placed in front of him. Technically the restraints could not be applied, and an injection could not be given, without a doctor's order. But who was really calling the shots?

This process was bluntly dubbed "shoot first and ask questions later" or simply "tie 'em up and shoot 'em up." It was also called "let 'em prove to us that they're okay to come out of restraints." The burden of proof lay with the patient. It might seem like a pathological need on the part of both nurse and doctor to control things, but the process of restraining and medicating a psychotic patient becomes a necessary and therapeutic step in the patient's treatment. Giving truly ill patients sedatives and antipsychotic medications allows them a chance to regain a piece of sanity—to tamp down anxiety, hallucinations, and paranoia.

George receives a large injection, the solubilized medications mixed into a single syringe and delivered via an eighteen-gauge needle into the upper outer quadrant of his left buttock, where the thick muscle can soak up all those good tranquilizers and get them on their way to his brain. Venous capillaries absorb the drug, the blood then transports it via circulatory branches to the inferior vena cava, upward to the right atrium of the heart, down to the right ventricle, then to the lungs to pick up oxygen, back to the left atrium, and then down to the left ventricle, which ejects the blood carrying the drug into the ascending aorta and carotids into the brain.

George's brain, with its dopamine, histamine, benzodiazepine, and GABA (gamma-aminobutryric acid) receptors receiving the signals, decelerates to a resting pace. Not down for the count, mind you, but it descends to a mild snooze. The blockade of the dopamine receptors in the limbic system begins to dissolve the man's psychotic symptoms. Biologically, it's complex. Phenomenologically, it's a cakewalk: man goes to sleep crazy; man wakes up calmer, if not saner.

As I was soon to discover, the medication process was perpetuated because Christina and a few of her peers had become pretty talented mental health clinicians by dint of their experience. And, of course, she was someone to be, if not feared, then at least approached with some caution. By then, several of my physician colleagues were streaming past me toward the meeting room. "Thanks for the doughnut," I say. "You know, Bo, this place reminds me of a bitter and twisted summer camp, and we're like the counselors."

"Oh, yes, honey, you are *so* right," he says.

"Or maybe something like a twenty-four-seven casino, and we're just like the blackjack dealers or the floorwalkers."

"It *is* kind of like that," says Bo. "And much, much more. You just wait and see, girl."

When I leave the meeting an hour and a half later, I see George the patient careening around in front of the triage desk, none the worse for wear. He has slept off his injection, and I'm sure a psych tech helped him pee into a urinal while he was in restraints. (They wouldn't let him piss himself in points. They weren't *that* mean.) And, frankly, it seems that George has woken up from the shot much less irritable and at least a bit less crazy. It did him no harm.

But does the end justify the means?

. . .

Just a few weeks later, I find myself in a minor power struggle with Christina over medicating a patient. For ten minutes, a young woman in a locked seclusion room, supposedly manic but maybe also high on something, yells nonstop, her volume escalating, and now and again screams at the top of her lungs: "Fuck you, you motherfuckers, why the fuck did you lock me up in here? I want a lawyer, I want to use the phone, I want a shower, you guys had no right to lock me up in this fucking room!"

Her caterwauling grabs the attention of Christina, the shift's charge nurse. "Paul, can't you do something about her yelling?" she asks me.

"Well, she is behind a locked door, and she's not going to be able to hurt anyone." I know that the legal standard for emergent involuntary medication circa 1992 (and today, in fact) is that of imminent danger.

The patient howls in a pitch reminiscent of an injured dog or a coyote. The content is similarly disturbing: "What are you guys? You are sadistic motherfuckers. Let me the fuck out of here right now. I mean it. I'm going to sue all of you mother-fuckers when I get out of here!"

"Lovely, isn't it?" Christina says to me tartly.

"Do you think she eats with that mouth?" I say. "But she is exercising her freedom of speech."

The woman's soliloquy is now punctuated by bloodcurdling screams, the type that hearkens back to the days of true bedlam— the era of wet blanket wraps, straitjackets, and hydrotherapy— before psychotropic medications arrived at the state asylums. You can almost see Frances Farmer if you close your eyes.

"Paul, it's time to give her a shot," Christina says.

"Now I know why I had to get a hearing test before I started this job," I joke. I'm stalling a bit. I don't like the screaming, but I don't really want to medicate the patient. It's not as if she's going to break the door down and come out and club us to death.

"But Paul, we shouldn't have to listen to this kind of abuse."

"I can tune it out," I say, "if I try to."

"Well, I can't," she says. "You can't be serious. Can't you see her jacking up the other patients?"

I look around me and, no, I really can't see that, but I do want to listen to what she has to say, since she's worked in psychiatry at this hospital for more than ten years. I can see how all the yelling might have an agitating effect on the other patients, but all in all, the clinic is reasonably under control right now. In fact, no one is in points, and only one other patient is in seclusion.

"We should put her ass down," says Christina. "She's been refusing meds."

"Hey, I'd rather not give her a shot," I say. "She isn't hurting anyone. Yes, it is annoying, but she can't scream forever. She's just sitting on her bed; she hasn't even pounded on the door."

"But Paul, she's also as psychotic as the day is long. She's not going to get better with tincture of time."

Sooner rather than later, the young woman gets up off the bed and starts banging on the door, progressively louder and louder. Even I can now see that she might at least hurt herself with this thumping. "Okay, okay," I say. "Let's do it. Call IP, and we'll give her the old-fashioned—droperidol five, Benadryl fifty. I'll write the order."

Things go smoothly as we get the hospital police to help us put her in restraints and give her the injection. After we leave the room, taking off our rubber gloves, the med nurse safely disposing of the needle, the patient's screeching continues unabated for another four minutes. Then, finally, silence descends on the room. I look through the little judas window and see the woman sleeping peacefully on her back. The snarl and grimaces have melted away after the delivery of the sedatives. Within ten minutes, since she is deeply asleep, we untie her four-point restraints. We leave her door unlocked. She crashes for another two hours and then is able to come out, take a shower, eat dinner, and use the phone. Though still a bit cranky and suspicious, the woman is able to cooperate with staff and navigate the complex peer relationships of the dayroom.

Later, in the staff room, the nurse comes up to me and says, "See, Paul, see how much better she's doing?"

"Yeah," I say, tentatively, "you're right." It's weird. I feel bad that I had to order the shot at all, *and* I feel bad that I didn't give it sooner.

"Of course I'm right," she says, only half joking. "All those goddamn laws and rights don't take into account that we have sick people here who need treatment. We can't just let 'em scream for days, you know."

There it is again, that us-versus-them theme. I wonder if I will ever put things so bluntly myself. I still have a lot to learn, but at least I'm one of *us* now and not one of *them*.

. . .

Why did I choose to work in psych emergency? Much of it had to do with a gut feeling that my style of thinking and relating on an interpersonal level with both patients and staff were tailor-made for the place. I wasn't obsessive enough to be a psychoanalyst or a researcher. I was a little too glib, a little too forthright, and far too much of a nonconformist, rebellious toward authority figures, to submit to the prevailing doctrines of either of American psychiatry's dominant paradigms: one rapidly rising, the biomedical explosion; the other gradually declining, Freudian psychoanalysis.

I wanted action. I wanted to see things evolving. I couldn't wait for several years of psychoanalysis to pass to see if my patient got significantly better. I couldn't wait for several years while slaving away at a research project just to see my name on a few articles and scrambling to ascend the academic staircase.

I wanted results, if not in the next five to ten minutes, at least in the next several hours. I wanted to say the calming words, right here, right now, and choose the ideal medication to soothe an agitated and psychotic patient, preventing him from winding up in points or slugging somebody, getting him started, I would hope, on the road to recovery. I wanted to wade into the messy domain of clinical psychiatry, which is all the more shattered and tattered in psych emergency. The place forces one to make a decision; not much dithering or second-guessing or ruminating can be tolerated. It forces one to rely on gut instincts and common sense.

The players on the scorecard, both staff and patient, change from day to day. They are part of an ever-changing but tightly bound social fabric that exists in the evanescent here-today-gone-tomorrow, outta-sight-outta-mind atmosphere that very nearly defines the place. That hectic turnover appealed to me from day one. The work appeals to folks whose temperaments combine an odd mixture of low-grade attention deficit disorder with a high tolerance, but a distinct need, for maximal stimulation. We are a subset of adrenaline junkies, a term often applied to ER doctors and nurses, paramedics, firefighters, and smokejumpers. Maybe we are the couch potatoes among adrenaline junkies.

My mentor, Dr. Bob Buckley, describes himself this way: "The sorry truth is that I'm pretty much other-oriented in terms of my motivation. Left to my own devices, I'll sit by myself and read books, not doing too much of any goddamn thing. But in the emergency room, I've always got something or someone up in my face. It means I get efficient and I get things done. I like that feeling."

I also liked the nearly impossible challenges, which gave me a chance to feel like I was working against all odds, with a chance to figuratively pull a rabbit out of a hat. I could put in my best effort and let the chips fall where they might. This was an antidote to my own perfectionism. Emergency psychiatry is messy.

. . .

"Dr. Linde, are you sure this patient is medically cleared?" asks the evening charge nurse. She has worked here a long time and is known to be cautious and conservative when it comes to medical issues. She is also known to be a bit on the nagging and controlling side as well. I've been told by my colleagues that, as a rookie attending psychiatrist, I will be tested by all the nurses, a process that could take at least six months.

"Yes," I say definitively. "I spoke with the ER attending, and it's all pretty straightforward. Dehydration, low potassium, both corrected."

"But the patient looks awful."

"Yes," I say. "He does. He's lost nearly twenty pounds, and he's in the midst of a probable psychotic depression, almost catatonic."

"Well, is he able to keep himself hydrated?" she asks.

A reasonable enough question. "I hope so," I say. "He was drinking juice in the ER."

"Are we sure that his failure to thrive is not due to an underlying medical illness, like cancer? I mean, a twenty-pound weight loss in a man in his fifties could be cancer. He looks terrible."

Jeez, anyone could have cancer and have it go undetected, I think. I find the question a little unfair and off the mark. I'm getting moderately impatient but decide to continue to allay her concerns. Kill her with kindness. "Well, his vital signs are okay. He's acutely stable. No one can say for sure whether or not he has an occult cancer brewing, but that can get sorted out when he's an outpatient or when he gets admitted."

"If it were my father or my uncle, then I'd really want him to at least get a chest x-ray."

I burst, just a little. "Listen, he's not in the midst of a medical emergency. It seems like you don't trust my medical judgment."

"Oh, doctor, no, of course I do," she says, half convincingly. "It's just those ER docs, they sometimes disregard our patients."

That's true, I think, but still she seems overly cautious. If I thought she was questioning me purely out of concern for the patient, then that would be one thing. But I feel she's pushing me to find out what my threshold for medical wellness in psych emergency is (reasonable enough), and just how much BS I can take, and how and if I will set limits (unreasonable, but human nature being what it is . . .).

"You know," I say, "I'll be here until 11 P.M. If he goes south, we can just ship him back."

"I hope so," she says. "You know how the ER can be about our patients, always dumping on us."

Yes, in my early days in PES, the relationship between psych emergency and the medical emergency department was acrimonious, to say the least. And the mistrust ran high. I sigh. "Yes, I know." I'm familiar with this anxious, catastrophist mind-set.

. . .

The nurses who gave me my informal orientation were trained, and had practiced for years, in an environment in which clinical decisions were made on the basis of a patient's need for treatment, at a time when state-of-the-art treatment was a combination of physical and chemical restraints for extremely disturbed patients. The nurses no doubt found that the new policies, regulations, and laws put a major dent in their ability to treat patients. They were accustomed to being in charge. They were not accustomed to deferring to a patient's wishes. "How can *that* one provide informed consent, Paul? *He's so crazy,*" Christina might say. And she'd be right.

The practice of acute care psychiatry at this time was not far removed from that of the era of rapid tranquilization, when the theory was that a veritable boatload of injected antipsychotic medication could somehow ablate symptoms of psychosis. "Titrate to stiff and drooling" was the motto. After you're injected with one hundred milligrams of Haldol, usually delivered into the gluteus but occasionally the thigh or the shoulder, yes, pretty much everything (in particular your consciousness) is obliterated.

Oh, how some of the more experienced nurses waxed rhapsodically about the good old days of rapid tranquilizing. The old antipsychotics, like Haldol, Prolixin, and Thorazine, were also called neuroleptics, medications that caused neurolepsy, a term that roughly means shutting your entire nervous system down—a sort of short-term but reversible mental and emotional paralysis also referred to as a chemical straitjacket or chemical restraint.

When I was an intern working in SFGH's inpatient psychiatric ward in 1989, just three years earlier, I could order an intramuscular backup, a shot, if a patient refused his oral dose of antipsychotic medications. This clinical approach was considered legal simply because the patient had been detained on an involuntary psychiatric hold. In other words, the patient did not retain the right to refuse psychiatric medications. The legal and ethical principles involved were presumed to rest on the reality that the patient was in need of treatment. The patient was deemed to be suffering from a treatable medical or psychiatric condition, and the system trusted the physician's judgment in deciding what treatment was most appropriate.

The notion, often referred to as paternalism in an ethical construct, is based on the concept of *parens patriae,* which was the standard for civil commitment until the late 1960s. This principle says that the state takes responsibility for people unable to care for themselves and identifies and treats patients on the basis of medical necessity or a need for treatment. Trusting the state was perhaps not as difficult then as it is now. *Parens patriae* presumed that the physician would act with beneficence and nonmaleficence even though this potentially interfered with a patient's autonomy.

According to the most authoritative textbook on American psychiatry, a patient's right to treatment was made paramount in the 1966 case *Rouse v. Cameron.* At the time, Judge David Bazelon noted that "the purpose of involuntary hospitalization is treatment and concluded that the absence of treatment draws into question the constitutionality of the confinement. Treatment in exchange for liberty is the logic of the ruling."[2] But by 1992, when I became an attending psychiatrist, I could give a patient involuntary medications only if I believed he posed an imminent danger to himself or others or if a court of law, presided over by a judge with no mental health training, had ruled that the patient was incompetent and did not retain the right to refuse treatment, which essentially referred to medications.

Case law stemming from a mid-1980s decision, *Riese v. St. Mary's,* in which a hospital was held liable for a patient's adverse reaction to medications received involuntarily, now directs hearing officers of the local mental health court to decide whether a patient is competent to refuse psychiatric medications. These are referred to as Riese hearings. To the hearing officer, the severity of the psychiatric illness is essentially irrelevant. What matters is whether the patient can state somewhat coherently what he or she doesn't like about the treatment's potential side effects or toxicity. If the patient can do so, or be coached to do so by his or her public defender, then the hearing officer frequently finds that the patient is sufficiently competent to refuse treatment.

Ultimately, it is a physician's mandate to alleviate suffering and provide treatment. What I know, and knew even back then, is that prompt, aggressive psychopharmacologic treatment at the beginning of a psychotic episode often puts an individual on track to get much, much better over the course of days to weeks.

When a nurse advocates giving a patient a shot, he or she knows that it might be the beginning of a longer course of treatment that may not only reduce immediate psychotic symptoms but also literally give the patient his or her life back. That's huge. Though it's often difficult to anticipate just how much better a patient will get with treatment, the improvement can be dramatic. And the psychiatric nurses with whom I worked were much, much closer, sometimes fifteen years closer, than I was to the days when patients' treatments were based on the idea that the patients were sick with a remediable illness. How could one blame a nurse for wanting to treat the sick?

TWO

THE ROOKIE

Bruno's Man Down

In the rear of a single cell, deep in the worst tier of a dilapidated county jail, a young man is found hanging. Within minutes, he's been transformed from a living, breathing man into 140 pounds of near lifelessness suspended nine feet above a concrete floor, his Nike-sneakered feet dangling. A knotted, jail-issued sheet stretches from a water pipe to the young man's puffy neck, the contours of his face obscured by swelling.

Once the hanging victim is found, the response is swift. Two burly officers hoist the inmate while a more nimble deputy works the edge of the linen with dull industrial-size scissors. After the victim has been plopped on a gurney, the jail nurses and I begin our resuscitation attempts.

The jail, for once, is eerily quiet. It's as if the young man's fellow inmates can sense the immediacy of the life-and-death battle that's just begun. I imagine they wait, hushed. Or maybe it's just that I've blocked out all the noise in order to perform the job that's ahead of me.

. . .

It's exactly one week before the hanging man is found in a cell on Six North of San Francisco County Jail #3—also known as San Bruno jail or just Bruno—that I pull Rollie Jefferson's chart from an overflowing file cabinet in the jail medical office. The jail psych notes are sparse but legible. Mitch, a jail social worker, had seen him and referred him to me for an antidepressant evaluation. I make a mental note that he's housed on Six North in a one-man cell, number 54, deep in the tier. After reviewing Mr. Jefferson's chart, I ride the gauntlet, climbing the stairs to see him in his cell. The staircase is visible to a significant number of inmates. As I reach the top, slightly out of breath, I spy a single deputy sitting on a chair, solely responsible at that moment for the more than two hundred of San Bruno's toughest customers located on that floor alone. "Hey, Deputy Martinez, how's it goin'?" I shout over the jail's never-ending bedlam.

"Not bad," answers Martinez, a fresh toothpick bobbing up and down in the corner of his mouth. "Not bad at all. Whaddya need?"

"I'm Dr. Linde, jail psych."

"Yeah, I remember you, doc."

"I'm here to see an inmate, Rollie Jefferson, cell 54, Six North."

"Just a second, let me check my custody roster. You know how they move these assholes around so much. Yup, there he is. Rollie Jefferson, single cell, 6-N-54."

"Why's he housed alone, deputy?"

"Let's look at his housing card, " says Martinez, one of Bruno's nicest and most experienced deputies, one I am glad to see. "Let's see, citizen Jefferson has been in some fights downtown, gang related, so they sent him out to Bruno, where, for some reason, we got less gang bullshit goin' on these days."

"So, do you know him at all?"

"Yeah," says Martinez. "I know him a little. He's on lock-down a lot, keeps him out of fights. We take him out for showers, exercise, chow. No problems from him. Kinda quiet. Do you want me to let you in, doc?"

"Um," I start. "Uh, I was hoping you could escort me in there." I am aware of the jail's "no hostage" policy. This means that, if I am kidnapped while interviewing the patient alone, the authorities will not negotiate with the inmate for my release. I think it prudent to prepare for the worst, and if I'm gonna be taken hostage, it may as well be with a strong and savvy deputy.

"Well, doc, I'm the only one up here on Six now—rest of the guys are at chow. Wait a second, and I can get somebody up from Four or Five to keep an eye on things." Martinez grunts into the radio, speaking rapidly in Spanish, his words punctuated by the squawking and static of the antiquated walkie-talkie system. Then, the response, unintelligible to me, comes in a stream of breathless Spanish. "Just a second, doc, my buddy's coming up from Five."

Once Deputy Rivera arrives, Martinez turns his oversized key in the lock, leading me into a dungeon of sorts. I stiffly walk past several inmates. Catcalls—"Hey, psych, hey, psych, you comin' to see me?"—follow me down the boulevard of incarceration. I peer forward, mumbling chitchat at Martinez. As the novelty of my appearance wears off, the hollering tapers, and inmates return to playing cards on concrete picnic tables or engaging in horseplay reminiscent of that of preteens at a playground. We stop in front of cell 54; nothing distinguishes it from its neighbors. Mr. Rollie Jefferson presents himself, lying in a supine position, as an elongated faceless lump under a rough bedcover. He demonstrates one of the inmate's many survival tricks—that of covering his face, eyes, and ears with his blanket—to speed the passing of time, to try to drown out the slammer's racket.

Martinez yells in, "Hey, Jefferson, psych here to see you. Rise and shine. Yo, Jefferson, up and at 'em, psych doc's here to see you!"

No answer from the form.

"Jefferson, no more sleeping beauty now," says Martinez. "The man here to see you. His time is important, so get your ass up!" The phrase "the man here to see you" reverberates through my head as I imagine a nineteenth-century plantation owner visiting his slaves in their hardscrabble lean-tos and shacks.

Martinez tumbles the lock, talking loudly to Mr. Jefferson all the time. The deputy shakes his shoulder. Mr. Jefferson's body doesn't budge. I take a few stabs at trying to rouse him. Finally, Martinez sticks his thumbnail into Jefferson's shin.

"Mothafucka, what the fuck is going on here?" Mr. Jefferson yells, springing to attention with sleepy eyes and a startled look on his face.

"Sorry to scare you, man," I offer.

"Nobody scares me," he growls.

"Okay," concedes Martinez. "Psych here to see you."

"I don't want to see no psych," replies Mr. Jefferson. He promptly lies back down and pulls his blanket over his head. "Go away. How about tomorrow?"

"I won't be here tomorrow," I say. "I'm here now."

His silence is deafening, even amid Bruno's encompassing commotion. "My name is Dr. Linde." I speak loudly to be heard over the tumult. "I am the psych who can prescribe medications for you. Mitch sent me to see you. I gotta talk to you to see if medicine might help you." I glance at my watch, obscured by the tattered edge of my jean-jacket sleeve. My appointment book shows a bulging list of ten, and on this night in San Bruno jail my tolerance for cajoling reluctant patients is marginal at best. I know that I can simply write "Inmate refuses eval" in Mr. Jefferson's chart and go on my merry way, so I'm not sure why I'm cutting him so much slack. "Mr. Jefferson, can you hear me?" I shout.

"Yessir!" comes the sarcastic response. "I *am* listening!"

"Okay," I say. "Sorry we woke you up. It's just that I'm only here one evening a week, and I wanted to talk to you for a little while to see if there's something I can do to help you. If you're interested, then you'll take those covers off your head, sit up, and swing your feet over to the floor so we can talk. If not, that's your choice. I'll give you five seconds."

"Uh, huh," comes a muffled response.

Martinez rocks on the soles of his feet, eyeing his own watch. "Hey, I got to get going. Rivera's due for a break."

"I only need a few minutes. Okay, Jefferson, listen up—five, four, three, two, one." More stillness from the figure. "Okay," I say, "we're out of here." As Martinez and I turn to leave, Mr. Jefferson sits bolt upright, flings off his covers, and swings his legs over the side of the bunk.

"All right, doc, I'm ready to talk to you 'bout some of your psycho-tropics," he says, the word's second half pronounced like the equatorial zone.

"You're lucky I'm a nice guy," I say, "or I'da been gone by now."

"Well, I'm not such a nice guy," says Martinez. "I've got to get back to the post. When you're done, doc, just close the cell door behind you. I'll let you out of the front of the tier."

"Thanks, Deputy Martinez." Standing deep in Six North, I feign courage and forge on: "Mitch sent me to see you because he was worried about you."

"Yeah, I'm worried about myself."

"How so?"

"I've been thinkin' a lot of bad thoughts, you know."

"About who? About what?" I sit down on the end of the bed.

"'Bout myself," explains Mr. Jefferson, his eyes seeming to study the laces of his beat-up court shoes. "Thinking that I'm bad, don't deserve to live, that I'm a piece of shit, 'scuse my language."

"Don't worry about it," I say. "I've heard worse. Does it ever get so bad that you think about killing yourself?"

"Oh, no, " he says, cracking into the slightest of smiles. "I'm not that down on myself, man."

"Have you ever thought about hanging yourself or shooting yourself or jumping off the bridge?"

"What you got me pegged for? A crazy man?" he says, bursting into a throaty, full-blown guffaw, smiling widely and clapping me on the shoulder, catching me off guard. "I ain't suicidal. I'm just stressed out. I'm not mothafuckin' crazy!"

"Of course you're not crazy, Mr. Jefferson. Would I be sittin' here on your bunk if I thought you wuz a mothafuckin' crazy man?" I take on the tone of a wanna-be-black suburban white kid, known on the streets as a "wigger."

"Hah, doc," he laughs, a gap-toothed grin showing. "You should be 'scusin' your language, too. But I do see your point."

. . .

Until the young man was discovered strung up by a twisted orange bedsheet in his cell, the evening, with its routine jail-house discomforts, must have seemed ordinary to the deputies on duty. Some things were taken for granted in the damp, dark version of hell called Bruno: the dank chill; deafening noise; the stench of overflowing toilets; holes in the concrete walls; scampering rats; bad institutional food; and the perpetual rattling of jailers' keys, reminiscent of the Great Depression.

The crumbling, outdated San Bruno jail had been constructed in the first half of the twentieth century on fog-shrouded land in the blue-collar town of San Bruno, ten miles south of the city. (Even then, San Francisco's available real estate and its incarcerated citizens lay in opposite directions.)

I usually arrived at Bruno about 6:30 P.M. on Thursdays. I'd be tired, hungry, and a bit fried after having worked a ten-hour day as a resident on the inpatient psych ward. Driving through the heavy iron gate marking the entrance to Bruno, I often observed a thick blanket of fog enveloping the decrepit six-story edifice. The chill was palpable. Often, as I drove the last hundred feet or so, I shivered, rolling up my car window, not knowing what was ahead. Even on a good shift, Bruno's atmosphere seemed to spring from the reels of a horror film.

I would ascend a massive stairway, visible to the inmates behind bars, in the midbelly of the building. The inmates were housed on the second through sixth floors. One or two deputies would be stationed on each floor. Two very long causeways, generally referred to as tiers, stretched away from the middle on each floor, one toward the north and the other toward the south. This explained the names of the tiers: Three South, Five North, and so on. These tiers, each with its own locked front gate, were lined with one- and two-man cells and extended nearly a football field's length away from the deputies. The officers thus were stationed far from the madness and mayhem deep on the tiers. For the humiliated, the sodomized, and the battered, it was too far away, literally and figuratively, from the civilized world.

As the floors went higher, the inmates generally got bigger, badder, and nastier. The tiers of Six North and Six South housed the most unruly inmates. On the second and third floors, the crime world's relative pussycats resided. The fourth floor was worse, and the fifth was a very close second to Six. The first floor consisted of administrative offices.

No matter the weather, I wore a jean jacket to work in the jail. I imagined that this layer of cloth, covering my rumpled dress shirt, somehow protected me from harm, a psychological talisman shielding me from the criminal element and the filthier layers of society.

I would walk up the stairs, located in the middle of Bruno, but in plain view of the throng of inmates who crowded the front of the tiers, closest to the deputies. As I trudged upward, I would always hear a similar refrain. "Hey, psych, you psych?" The name *psych* refers generically to all psychiatric staff in the jail. The shouts, good-natured, would get rolling. I would continue stepping, doing my best to ignore this mild hazing. "Hey, psych, I'm gonna kill myself, psych, whaddya gonna do about it?" Nice but not stupid, I rapidly learned to not take these jamming—slang for "manipulative"—hollow threats too seriously. In this situation, it was important to never make eye contact with the ersatz supplicants.

"You can't just walk past me. I'm gonna K-EEE-LL myself. You can't let me K-FEE-LL myself." Hearing this, I often thought,

"Just watch me, turkey," after which I would quicken my stride and hunch my shoulders, concentrating hard to fix my gaze straight ahead. The shouts would follow me: "Hey, psych, where you goin'? You can't let me K-EEE-LL myself!" Safely at a distance, I would usually sneak a peek back. Reassuringly, I usually saw the afflicted "patient" with a half dozen buddies huddled around him, laughing uproariously.

An ambient wall of sound—present morning, noon, and night at Bruno—ripped along at seventy decibels on the third floor but amped up to more than a hundred on the sixth floor. Word had it that the joint got quiet only between three and six in the morning, when even the manics took a short nap. I hoped to never find out for sure.

In this moonlighting gig during the early 1990s, I earned about $150, before taxes, for four hours of work. If I chose to cheat on my time sheet, I could make that much money for two and a half or three hours of work. Sometimes I felt entitled to a "bad karma, good business" surcharge because, instinctively, I knew that the work was shortening my life and polluting my outlook.

My working in the jail as a resident made me feel like a tough guy, bold and decisive. Sometimes wrong, but never in doubt. My jail mentor was a swashbuckling psychiatrist, Dr. Pablo Stewart, a bilingual Spanish-speaking Vietnam veteran who carried himself with the swagger of a surgeon and who, at the time, ran the forensic psychiatric ward at San Francisco General Hospital. Not coincidentally, I signed up for my gonzo jail doc job with two of my best friends: fellow second-year colleagues with hard-consonant one-syllable nicknames, burly, beer-drinking ex-jocks born and raised, like me, in America's flyover zone and new to town. Machismo! Bravado! Man up, hombre!

I worked Tuesday evenings at San Francisco's downtown lockup, the Waldorf by comparison, and Thursday evenings at Bruno. At the time, I possessed a young man's cowboy mentality. I was also naive. I had an adolescent-like feeling of relative invincibility. I figured, "Hey, I'm such a good guy, these inmates would never hurt me." In fact, I sometimes went up and evaluated prisoners on the tiers, interviewing them through the bars, sacrificing their confidentiality and my safety. My appearance as someone who seemed to care gave me a perfect line with which to let inmates off the hook gently.

The salty forensic psychologist orienting me gave me this advice within a half hour of meeting me: "You come across as a nice guy," he said. "If you're getting jammed for something, try this: Pretend you're talking with someone at a cocktail party. Make your decision about what you're gonna do inside of your head. If it happens to be what they want, then your job is easy. If you're gonna turn 'em down, then tell 'em with your most sincere face forward: 'I couldn't possibly let you take Sinequan. I care too much to let you take that stuff. It can cause heart failure. Really, it's for your own good that I won't prescribe you Sinequan.' And then get the hell out of there fast, before the psychopath figures out that he's been beaten at his own game." Many of the inmates who had been up to "the pen," often San Quentin or Vacaville, had become accustomed to a whopping nightly dose of Sinequan, the most soporific of the tricyclic antidepressants. In those days, it was handed out like candy to hardcore cons to dummy them up for at least twelve of the twenty-four hours of the day. Many inmates, used to shooting smack or drinking vodka or gobbling Valiums or smoking big bowls of weed on the outside, enjoyed the pharmaceutical hammer. And the guards liked this practice because it made the joint quieter, laying out bad guys, preventing them from stirring up shit on the tiers.

I often asked myself in those days: "What the hell am I doing here, namely, working in jail?" In fact it provided a sort of trial by fire. The opportunity to evaluate inmates as a neophyte was exhilarating, even sanctifying. Going it alone in the jail two evenings a week schooled me in the nuances of psychopathology, psychiatric diagnosis, substance abuse, psychopharmacology, the criminal subculture, and, for lack of a better term, suffering.

I'm embarrassed to admit now that, at the time, instead of feeling compassion for the inmates, what I felt most vividly was fear mixed with disgust. This was tempered by the stomach-churning thrill I felt upon entering the jail, enjoying my role as an observer of society's disasters and as someone who could mix it up with genuine bad guys, albeit in a controlled environment.

Yet when I sat down next to an affiliated gang member or career criminal, my heart pounded a little harder, a little faster, with a cold sweat sometimes not too far behind. The problem with working in a jail is that your fears based on things like skin color, hairstyle, or tattoos are amplified by the simple fact that many of the inmates, regardless of ethnicity, *are* relatively dishonest, cruel, and unafraid to commit crimes to survive in life.

· · ·

"So, Mr. Jefferson, do you ever think about just wishin' you were dead—like you just went to sleep and didn't wake up?"

"Want me to be honest with you?" Mr. Jefferson is intent again, his arms folded across his chest, his eyes focused on his tapping foot.

"Of course."

"You're not gonna lock me up in one of those rubber rooms, are you?"

"Oh, no, no way, no reason to do that," I say, which I mean, since he has already denied to me any sort of active suicidal ideation. But even at this stage of my career, I know a dirty little secret—it's always the psychiatrist's prerogative to change his or her mind.

"Okay, you're sure then?" he asks.

"Scout's honor," I say.

"Doc, truthfully, sometimes I lay up in the bed in the middle of the night, three o'clock, four o'clock, wide awake. It finally gets quiet in here about then, 'cept for all the snorin', course, and my mind does go to wanderin' about—what have I done with my life? Bein' a gangsta and all. The youngsters comin' up got no sense of honor, no respect for their elders. My grandmother raised me up a Baptist; we wuz taught that suicide is wrong. For all of the bad things that I've done, you know, I still go to church, I still believe in God. Grandmama put the fear of God into me. I wouldn't ever commit suicide. But if God were here tonight in this cell, you know, about four o'clock, if he could put me to sleep and take me, that'd be okay with me."

I'm struck by the pain in his voice, his sincerity. I wait before responding, my eyes falling to the floor, my face taking on a more serious frame. "So you're feelin' that bad, huh, Mr. Jefferson?"

"Yessir. Plus, I'm afraid to tell you this next part because you are sure enough gonna think that I am some kind of a crazy man."

"Listen, Mr. Jefferson, I might look young, but I've already seen a few hundred crazy guys in my career. I can tell you already that you're not crazy, you're just under a lot of pressure and you're trying to deal with it. There's a big difference."

"Thanks, doc," says Mr. Jefferson, pausing. "Sometimes in the middle of the night, when things get quiet, my grandmama comes to visit me. Right here in this cell, she comes right in and sets herself down on the bed, 'bout where you're sittin', and just sits there, smiling peacefully, looking at me."

"How long does she stay here?" I ask casually, knowing that such visions and visitations are not all that uncommon among people who are grieving the death of a loved one.

"Only a few seconds, ten maybe," he says.

"Does she say anything?"

"She's smiling, she's looking at me, her lips move, but I can't hear anything," he says, his voice lowering, his eyes looking directly into mine for the first time. "It's like a time warp when she comes, like time stops and everything gets even more quiet."

"When did your grandmama pass?"

Mr. Jefferson's face turns ashen. He holds back tears before speaking. "A week from tonight, 'bout this time, it'll be exactly one year ago."

"So, of course, it'll be the anniversary of her death," I say, highlighting for him and myself just how risky and painful the marking of time from a loved one's death can be. "One of the hardest days of a man's life."

"Really?" he says. He tries hard to stop the flow of tears. He rubs his eyes and inhales quickly before putting his hands over his face, hanging his head and holding it as if he has a headache.

"You may not be ready to cry in front of me, but you sure as hell should feel okay crying when you're alone. You've got a world of hurt on your head."

"Thanks, doc, I feel better just talkin' about it." He lifts his head and looks me in the eye.

"Good," I say. "A little of that can go a long way. The more you can talk about that with Mitch or with family, then the better you'll feel." I pause. "Now we should figure out whether you should take medication."

"I'd rather not," he says. "I've been going to meetings. See, I'm an addict, and I don't want to take anything if I don't have to."

"Of course not," I explain, "but these medications are different. They're prescribed by a doctor. They're not addicting. Depression is a medical condition, like diabetes or high blood pressure. It can be treated."

Generally, psychiatrists save the use of antidepressant medications for bona fide cases of major depression. In a place like the jail, an inmate's sleep, appetite, and energy are almost always adversely affected, rendering an assessment of the so-called physical symptoms of depression unreliable in making the diagnosis.

Sure enough, his sleep is poor, but his appetite and energy are fairly good. His concentration is off. Mr. Jefferson does acknowledge sadness about being locked up and the anniversary of his grandmother's death. He does suffer from a negative opinion of himself. Otherwise, he feels hopeful about rebuilding his life after jail by going back to school and getting a "nine-to-five." He tells me that he has earned his props as a longtime, high-ranking gang member, and that, if he made the decision to "retire" from the life, his decision would be respected. He enjoys basic things like listening to music and reading. He denies feeling guilty and recognizes that his grandmother raised him the right way and that it's time to set things straight on the outside.

"Well, Mr. Jefferson, you're in luck," I say. "I don't think you'll need medication, you don't have what we might call a clinical depression. I think your feelin' bad has to do with your stress level, especially because of your grandmama's death. It'll be important to talk with your family about it. Anybody come to mind?"

"Yeah, doc, I talk to my brother every other day on the pay phone. We're tight. We can talk about this."

"I also think some counseling from jail psych will help. How well do you get along with Mitch?"

"Oh, Mitch is cool. He listens to me, you know."

"Good. I'll make sure that he follows up with you this week. I'm afraid I'm gonna have to be movin' on. I got other people to see, but first I wanted to clarify something." I look Rollie Jefferson in the eye and ask him, "Can you promise me that you won't do anything to hurt yourself, that you won't commit suicide?"

He returns the look. "Truthfully, I can say that. I feel better. I think I'm gonna be okay."

"I'm glad to hear it. Unfortunately, I gotta run. Nice to meet you, Mr. Jefferson." I hold out my hand and he gives it a tight squeeze, not hostile but heartfelt.

"Hey, doc, one more thing. When are you comin' back to see me?"

I'm a little ashamed that I hadn't told him right off that this would be a one-shot evaluation, a point that, subsequently, I added to all of my jailhouse introductions. "The only people I see here regularly are those who I start on medications. Unless Mitch wants me to reevaluate you for medications, I won't be seeing you again. Mitch is a professional counselor; he can definitely help you with this stuff."

"I know, it was just I kinda like the way you put things. Thanks for your help."

"You're welcome, Mr. Jefferson. Good luck. I gotta close this door behind me, you know."

"I know."

After I close the door and start to the front of the tier, he yells after me: "Hey, psych, thank you! Thank you very fucking much!" As he says that, he laughs loudly, surveying his Six North associates in incarceration.

As I make my way to Martinez, buried in my jean jacket and in my thoughts, I try to figure that last thing out. The simple explanation is that he needs to display a "who gives a fuck?" attitude for his peers. But I also wonder if he isn't angry with me because I made a brief connection with him and got him in touch with some heavy emotions, and now he feels that I am abandoning him. I don't know.

. . .

The next Thursday night, a week after I had seen Rollie Jefferson and nine other unfortunates, I enjoy a fairly easy night, seeing only five inmates. I sit and do my charting in the tiny jail psych office, working at a metal desk covered with an unruly pile of papers. As I write my last note and prescription, I hear a quiet "Man down" squawk over the radio. I stop scribbling and listen more closely, not knowing the location of the call.

I know that attempted suicides on the tiers sometimes turn into man-down situations. My mind races. Could that man down be Rollie Jefferson? I instantly consider his suicide risk as the radio grows quiet for a moment. No history of suicide attempts. From Mitch's notes, I know that there's no family history of suicide. Looking at three more months in Bruno and then on probation. Plans to stay clean and sober, get married, and get a job working in construction for his future brother-in-law. My brief reverie is hijacked by the next radio call.

"Man down! Six North! Man down! Six North! All available medical personnel to the sixth floor. NOW!!!"

I don't always respond to man-down calls, but as the only physician in the house, albeit a green psychiatrist-in-training, I know this one is the real deal. I wheel out of my office on the first floor, adjacent to the jail's medical clinic, only to meet one of my favorite nurses, Victor, who is fairly sprinting to the staircase. I catch up to him. We hit the steps at a quick jog. Two of his colleagues, the ready-steady evening charge nurse, Marie, and the wacky but kindhearted Teri, prepare the rudimentary crash cart in the hallway before trundling it into an ancient iron elevator, which, unfortunately, moves at a glacial pace to the sixth floor. "Damn, Victor, doesn't sound good," I say. "Know who it is?"

"Don't know anything," he says, "except the lieutenant called 911 a couple minutes ago. A bad sign. Last 911 call a guy died of an MI."

"Hope it's not a suicide, not one of ours," I grunt, out of breath, realizing that my three-mile jogs in the park are not enough to keep me in tiptop shape.

Victor and I say nothing else as we run up the staircase, our fatigue and fear apparent to the strangely quiet inmates pressed to the front of their tiers as we tear past the third, fourth, and fifth floors on our way to the sixth. In a true rarity, the gates to

Six North are open, with a beefy deputy standing guard. Breathless, we sprint past a lineup of men in orange standing silently on either side of the tier. They stand almost at attention, uncharacteristically respectful, seeming to either know or sense the gravity of the situation deeper on the block. It's Jefferson, I think, panicking.

I stop dead in my tracks while Victor races ahead. Moments later, he turns around and yells at me, "Hey, get your ass up here, doc. I'm gonna need your help."

I don't really hear Victor, but I continue to walk slowly forward, as if in a dream. As I get closer, whew, I can see that the hubbub is around cell 52. Rollie Jefferson remains on lockdown in the cell next door. His hands wrapped around the vertical bars, he watches the proceedings. His face is a blank. "Hey, Rollie, you're alive!" I scream.

"Yeah, doc, but you need to help this other dude . . . and quick," he says.

The man down is technically a man *up*. As the deputies work to get him down, Victor and I stand numbly by. I feel helpless. One veteran GP describes this emotion well: "I believe every doctor has a secret 'what the hell am I doing here?' button hidden away in his psyche. Some emergencies seem unsolvable."[1]

"How long's he been up?" I ask, breaking out of my temporary daze, directing my question to Sergeant Ransom, who appears to be in charge of the scene, directing traffic and monitoring the progress of his three underlings.

"Don't know for sure, but some of the guys say it could have been as much as twenty minutes," explains Ransom, a tall and muscular black man, his graying beard and silver wire-rims giving him a distinguished appearance. "Last guy to talk to him was Milliken over there. Said it had been twenty minutes or more. Didn't notice anything different about him."

"Sure hope it's not one of our guys," I say, referring to our roster of psych clients incarcerated at Bruno.

"Doubt DuShane's one of yours," says Ransom. "Only been up here a couple days from downtown. Housing card says, per classification, no psych contacts, been in jail a month already."

Sergeant Ransom and I pause to look at the jailhouse photo on the front of the blue card. His fade haircut, goatee, and frown initially suggest another young black man trying to look tough. His date of birth suggests he is only eighteen. "Just a kid, Sarge," I say. "How'd he get housed up here?"

"Don't know," exhales Ransom as we once again watch Deputy Kingston hacking away at the sheet.

I try not to look too closely into the face of death. Kenneth DuShane's current countenance looks nothing like the kid in the jailhouse photo. Despite his attempt to look menacing, Kenneth DuShane's face in the photo is that of a teen who may have sat behind you in church or waited on your table at a local restaurant or played hoops in the neighborhood schoolyard.

Now, in his time of dying, he shows no wisp of innocent facial hair below his lower lip. No multilayered haircut. No, now his chin and scalp are clean-shaven. The hanging has transformed a youthful visage into a macabre mask, its features nearly obliterated by extensive swelling, tinged an eerie pale blue on a man whose visible arms and ankles are a deep mahogany.

Victor and I continue to stand by. We fidget as we wait for the deputies to cut him down, a seeming eternity, giving us time to divide the labor that Kenneth DuShane's attempted resuscitation will entail. Victor, an experienced medical-surgical nurse, will handle the ventilation and I will thump the chest, providing a measly circulation, 20 percent of the normal output of the heart. In these situations, I prefer the physicality and relative mindlessness of leaning over, pressing on the breastbone of the victim in an attempt to recapitulate the heart's pumping. The discharge of energy helps me handle my anxiety.

Although the night is cool and the fog's moisture permeates the place, I feel beads of sweat on my forehead and the unmistakable smell of my own body emanating from my armpits. Fight or flight. Victor breathes an audible sigh of relief when Marie and Teri arrive with the cart, which supplies us with a face mask and a balloonlike Ambu bag to make the process of ventilating Mr. DuShane safer and more efficient.

Finally the deputies finish their work. Kenneth DuShane is dumped face-up on a gurney that Teri and Marie hustled up from the medical office.

Airway? No doubt blocked to some extent by soft tissue swelling. Breathing? No way. Circulation? Extremely doubtful, but, out of habit, I finger the man's neck to check his carotid pulse. The flesh feels odd to me—buoyant but firm at the same time. I also feel his wrist to check his radial pulse. Of course there is none. The most we can do is ventilate him with 100 percent oxygen delivered from a green tank by tubing it into the Ambu bag as I pound his chest rhythmically with the heel of my hand until the San Mateo County paramedics arrive.

I take to doing the compressions five times, then waiting for ventilatory support in the form of Victor squeezing the Ambu bag, the air rushing through a short tube and into the clear plastic face mask tightly sealed around Mr. DuShane's mouth, before I continue. As Victor squeezes, I pause and stand back, duly noting DuShane's chest rise as a rush of air enters his lungs.

When Marie checks the femoral artery, she tells me that she feels a faint pulse with each of my compressions. When she presses her stethoscope to Mr. DuShane's chest, she tells me that she hears a reassuring whoosh of air each time Victor squeezes the Ambu bag.

The fact that Victor and I make a good team, giving our best effort, provides little consolation. I know that if Mr. DuShane survives, he is going to be a vegetable. Death seems merciful in comparison. But the inside of a jail cell, in the heat of the moment, is not, for me, a place for contemplation. It is a place for action. At the time, getting a heartbeat feels like all that matters.

Looking up from my work, I notice something strange. The deputies allow about five or six orange-clad inmates to stand silently in a semicircle just outside the door to DuShane's cell. They mumble softly to one another.

The ten minutes before the paramedics arrive seem an eternity, but eventually they charge through the gates of hell. I have never been so relieved to relinquish responsibility. I watch them work as I lean against the filthy wall, my jean jacket protecting me from germs and insanity perhaps, but not from death. My forehead exudes sweat despite the ambient coolness.

The paramedics work, guided by radio transmissions from an ER doc at Seton Medical Center, "Our Lady of 280," a Catholic hospital perched above a busy metropolitan loop freeway. They seem to be sweating it a bit. Here is a young hanging victim, without a pulse and breathless, facial features obliterated by swelling, who is laid flat on a jailhouse gurney in a scene out of *Cool Hand Luke*.

The surrounding inmates continue to act as witnesses. The paramedics rapidly and skillfully intubate the young man. The Ambu bag works nicely in delivering oxygenated air to his lungs. The paramedics pump powerful cardiac medications into his intravenous line. They shock his heart electrically.

The smallest flicker of hope, the beginning of the end, emerges when one of the paramedics spots a minuscule but tangible blip on the EKG monitor. The tracing slowly enlarges, but it is clearly abnormal. The intermittent electrical firing of the heart muscle results in a very weak pulse. With this relatively good news, I see the paramedics getting antsy. I'm sure they want to take the kid out of here breathing and with some sort of pulse, even the puny one now registering on the monitor.

Suddenly, the paramedics give Sergeant Ransom a sort of a high sign, and they quickly pack up all their gear, switch the gurney wheels from "lock" to "spin," and start hauling ass out of there. The semicircle of inmate witnesses turns around, but they stand their ground like the guards in front of Jesus's tomb on Easter morning. The rest of the inmates gather on either side of the tier, looking almost reverential, speaking to one another in hushed tones. You could put suits, topcoats, wingtips, and fedoras on them, and they would look like any other group of stunned mourners standing at attention next to an open gravesite as the first shoveled clods of dirt hit the shiny top of a casket.

Victor and I jog absentmindedly behind the departing paramedics. I, the lone physician, a medically unseasoned second-year resident, a psychiatrist-in-training, helpless in the face of a potentially preventable death, follow the seemingly omniscient and omnipotent paramedics. We hit the elevators and trundle down, eventually making our way out the front door of the jail.

I then watch the paramedics transfer a most certainly brain-dead Kenneth DuShane into the back of a county ambulance. It speeds off silently, its red light flashing—the bulb getting progressively dimmer as the vehicle disappears into a thick nighttime fog.

· · ·

Kenneth DuShane never regained consciousness in the intensive care unit of Our Lady of 280. Despite the fact that his body did get intubated, ventilated, and resuscitated, his badly damaged, oxygen-deprived heart simply stopped working.

No one knows when his figurative heart gave out. He hanged himself either after a period of contemplation and premeditation, or simply impulsively.

To my knowledge, no psychological autopsy was performed on Mr. DuShane. Obviously, I never talked to him before he died. But I have evaluated dozens of men of a similar demographic. Epidemiological studies would suggest that, because he was a young black male, his suicide risk was greater than that of the average person. In addition, he likely felt alienated and isolated. Maybe his girlfriend had just broken up with him. Maybe he had just been sentenced to the penitentiary. Maybe he suffered from a drug problem. Maybe his parents had abused or neglected him. I don't know.

The letter of commendation that I received from San Bruno's commanding officer, Captain Koehler, could not bring Kenneth DuShane back. His heart had been broken, his body rendered useless. I would like to think that his spirit, decimated in life, escaped and ascended with his soul. I want to believe that his spirit traveled upward through the mist blanketing San Bruno jail that night, departing at precisely the moment that his shell of a body was touched by the cool night air, under the watch of a forgiving God.

THREE

THE SCRAMBLER

How to Prevent a Murder

When I was a third-year resident in psychiatry, Sal Pauletti was referred to me for an evaluation by his primary care doctor, who wrote, "Mr. P. is a 50-year-old Vietnam War veteran with PTSD [post-traumatic stress disorder], possible psychotic disorder and a history of migraine headaches with no ongoing psych treatment. Married with a stable occupation. He complains of conflicts with his boss. He reports violent tendencies, troubles with impulse control."

Prior to seeing the patient, I call his internist, Dr. Jesus Ramirez, a brand-new attending physician and the source of the referral. I run the gauntlet of receptionist, nurse, and physician's assistant rapidly, but not because I am a fellow physician. No, it seems that our common patient's name rings a bell in the minds of those health care workers as each one, in turn, picks up the phone receiver.

"Oh, yes, of course, right away," each one says. "You're the psychiatrist."

Such deference for a psychiatrist among nonpsychiatric health care professionals is usually correlated with a great clinical need for your help with a certain patient. It's also a rough indicator of the patient's difficulty. Generally it's not a good sign.

I know Jesus slightly from his last couple of years spent as a resident on call. We had shared in the collective misery of being house officers together in our post-medical-school training. He is a tall, husky, jovial guy known for his sound medical judgment and levelheadedness under fire.

"Hi, Dr. Ramirez," I start, "this is Paul Linde. I'm a third-year psych resident here at UC, and I'm scheduled to see Sal Pauletti, the patient you referred for a psych eval. I don't know if you remember me, but I'm pretty sure we've met a few times in the hospital."

"Oh, hi, Paul, of course," he says. "How are things going?"

"Not bad," I say, "except for this referral."

I hear a long, loud sigh on the other end of the line. "Yeah, Paul, there's more to the story than I could put in writing. He told me he wanted to kill his boss, maybe kill his wife, maybe himself. I thought it might be time for you guys to get involved."

"Yeah, no doubt about it," I say. "Danger to self, danger to others, the whole shebang."

"Medically, there's not much going on. He has hypertension and is on Zestril. He used to be an alcoholic and a drug addict, but claims he's been clean and sober for almost twenty years. He was telling me about his problems with anger, and, well, stupid me, I asked him if he could give me an example."

"No," I say. "Good job of screening."

"And this question opened up a can of worms—he told me he was angry with his boss at work and was thinking about killing him. What freaked me out most was how calm he was when he was telling me about it."

"How's he feel about seeing a psychiatrist?"

"He's okay with it," says Jesus. "Maybe even a little too eager."

"So, when did you see him last?" I ask.

"Last Friday." A pause. "And they got him in to see you already?" he asks.

"A high perceived need, I would say. He's scheduled to see me tomorrow at two o'clock," I reply.

"Wow, that's quick."

"Well, it sounds like he needs it. I'll see what I can do. I'll give you a call tomorrow or the next day and fill you in."

. . .

Sometimes it's good to not know what you don't know. Before my first solo office visit with a homicidal maniac, a much-feared but seldom-encountered psychiatric patient, I didn't even come close to realizing any of the things that I did not know. According to the forensic psychiatrist Robert Simon, the author of *Bad Men Do What Good Men Dream,* the follow ing statements are true: "Psychiatrists have long known that the most dangerous time is during the first visit with an unknown patient. According to an American Psychiatric Association Task Force Report, 40% of psychiatrists are assaulted during their careers. Nearly three-fourths of assaults against all physicians occurred during the first meeting of doctor and patient."[1] I wonder why none of my supervisors ever informed me of these facts. Maybe they didn't know. Maybe they didn't think it was important. Maybe they didn't want to alarm me. Or maybe they were operating under their own well-tailored cloaks of denial.

I approached this evaluation with little fear—maybe a little performance anxiety to temper my boredom. But in psychiatry, as in life, sometimes destiny deals you a joker from the pack.

. . .

It's Thursday afternoon. I look at the cheap clock on my desk and see that it's a couple minutes before two o'clock. I breathe a heavy sigh, wishing I had a window in my eight-foot-by-eight-foot office, the spartan setup reflecting my rank in the Department of Psychiatry's food chain. I once again read the consultation request, not recognizing the danger lurking within it.

I get up and slowly walk down the hallway toward a dimly lit waiting room. I silently stop just outside the door to see if anyone is there. I see a man sitting, slumped, reading an old *Popular Mechanics*. That must be him. He does not seem to notice me, so I spend a few moments watching him before I speak.

"Mr. Pauletti?"

The man flinches, nearly leaping out of his seat.

"I'm Dr. Linde," I say, stepping inside and extending my hand for him to shake.

He gathers himself, stands up, brushes himself off, and nods to me, saying nothing, quickly jamming his hands in his pockets.

"Please follow me," I say flatly. After a few steps, I slow my pace, now only a step or two ahead, glancing over my shoulder furtively, briefly, to try and size up this guy in a preliminary fashion. As the wise guys of psychiatry are fond of saying, the evaluation starts right away.

Sal Pauletti is not a physically imposing man, standing little more than five feet seven inches tall and weighing not much more than 160 pounds. He wears a Mets cap pulled down low over his forehead, his eyes seeming to study the floor in front of him as he walks. He looks anxious, but I sense little to no menace in his manner, appearance, or behavior. He raises not even a transient flicker in my gut check for violence potential, a product of the limbic system and primitive cortex of *Homo sapiens*. This gut feeling is an evolutionary holdover from caveman days and, surprisingly, is the psychiatric clinician's most accurate barometer of potential violence at a moment's notice.

We enter my office, and I point to a utilitarian chair designated for patients and begin to settle into my similarly mundane chair, which faces him. The quarters are cramped, and it's a tad warm and stuffy. Tacky Impressionist paintings and my med school diploma adorn the walls. He readily sits. Our feet nearly touch, just a couple of feet apart.

But before I can utter a word, Mr. Pauletti surveys my office, his eyes scanning the scene rapidly, and stands up abruptly. Perplexed, I can only watch as I see him escalate into a state of agitation, still saying nothing, his feet shuffling as he begins to systematically tap all four of my office walls, rapping his knuckles softly but purposefully up, down, and all around.

I am flabbergasted. I hadn't come across this situation before, even in the inpatient psych ward or the emergency room. Is he looking for monitoring devices? Could he be that paranoid? He breathes loudly, huffing faster and faster. Is it a panic attack? He's a combat vet. Could it be a flashback? I watch him—more with a sense of curiosity than fear. As his behavior persists, however, I begin to feel more afraid. Is he going to physically explode? Is he having a stroke, a seizure?

My heart begins to race. Having to discard my customary introduction and explanation—the things I would normally say to a patient at our first meeting—I become even more anxious. Though I have worked with plenty of agitated patients before, the setting has always been much more secure—with colleagues, nurses, and psych techs around and police officers readily available if things got really rough. I do my best to stay calm. I show no fear. It is pure improvisation on my part. I'm churning intellectually and emotionally, hoping that things do not escalate into a physical scramble. I'm in survival mode, relying on my wits instead of any great experience or knowledge of the human mind.

Mr. Pauletti continues rapping his knuckles on the walls, hyperventilating. At a certain point, I can stay silent no longer. "Whoa, Mr. Pauletti, are you okay, man? You look a little messed up. Nervous. Is there something I can do to help you?"

He glares at me. His breathing noticeably slows; his fists unclench; his mouth stays closed; his gaze drops to the floor; and he slowly sits down. He suddenly grabs a coffee mug off my desk and swings it in the air slowly from side to side, his stare vacant. After a few moments, he laughs to himself and sets the cup down.

I breathe again.

He still says nothing, but seems to calm down even more. He pushes the brim of his cap up, exhaling, sweating like he has just finished boxing a couple of rounds. His feet stop moving; his hands slowly come to rest in his lap. Sweat drips off the tip of his nose and a band of moisture soaks the headband of his cap. Rings of sweat stain the armpits of my white oxford dress shirt. I loosen my tie. "So what's going on, Mr. Pauletti?" I ask, trying very hard to sound nonchalant, using a regular-guy "hey buddy" approach with him. It is as if I'm trying to tame a Tasmanian devil.

He slowly readjusts his gaze, his eyes moving up until they are locked onto mine. He appears to me as one who is emerging from a period of blindness.

"Are you sure you want to know?" The words ooze out of his mouth.

I waste no time in replying. "Yes, Mr. Pauletti, yes, of course."

"I'm planning to kill my boss," he says casually, as if he were telling me his date of birth or his shoe size.

Yikes, I think, trying mightily to keep my cool. I'm attempting to convey a sense of "No big deal, pal, I deal with homicidal maniacs every day." Although my regular-guy approach calms him, his statement opens a Pandora's box.

"And I know a way to do it so that I would never be caught," he adds, barely missing a beat.

Already trained in the way a psychiatrist should stereotypically respond when presented with intensely disturbing information, I say nothing, peer down at my hands, and absentmindedly clear my throat before once again looking him in the eye. I see that his liquid brown eyes are bloodshot from God knows what. My thoughts swim with fear and mild panic.

"No one else knows, not even my wife."

I stifle my natural inclination to say something, even "Uh-huh," to mask my nervousness. I have been taught to let the opening moments of any clinical encounter unfold organically, with the patient taking the lead. Some supervisors said the more silence, the better. This approach is in distinct opposition to my instinct, which is to start chatting, to somehow dissolve the rising tension in the room. At the time I even think, What the hell? Why not say nothing? I don't know what to say, anyway.

Just then, a brain wave saves me: Oh, yes, that's right, think risk assessment. Think the basics; play cub reporter; act dispassionately; find out what, where, when, why, and how. I mentally review the basics of performing what's called a violence risk assessment.

. . .

Simon may have written that the "ability of mental health professionals to predict violence is a myth,"[2] but I'm still obligated to try to tease out the risk factors. From a medicolegal perspective, the first thing I'm expected to do is calculate the patient's acute risk of perpetrating violence. To perform this task, I must harness the power of every one of my neurons, many of them operating, no doubt, in my subconscious.

In his book *Blink,* Malcolm Gladwell writes, "I think that this is the way that our unconscious works. . . . It's sifting through the situation in front of us, throwing out all that is irrelevant while we zero in on what really matters. And the truth is that our unconscious is really good at this, to the point where thin-slicing often delivers a better answer than more deliberate and exhaustive ways of thinking."[3]

Only two risk factors consistently show up in the assessment of the risk of violence. The first is the use of alcohol or other drugs, and the second is a history of perpetrating violence. Otherwise, the risk factors that predispose an individual to violence compose a commonsensical laundry list: the individual makes threats; has a plan to commit violence, with both the intention of and means for violence; has a history of poor impulse control or antisocial behavior; is experiencing overt stressors or losses; is young, male, poor, and socially isolated; is paranoid; has a history of vandalizing; has access to weapons; experiences command auditory hallucinations; or has severe mood or personality disorders.

To discharge my professional duty, I have to at least try to find out the name, address, and phone number of Mr. Pauletti's boss. I also need to find out just what Mr. Pauletti has in mind for the, ahem, disposition of his boss. I tell myself to take measures to protect the boss and, of course, help Mr. Pauletti prevent himself from acting on his homicidal plans—a path that could lead to prison or the morgue for him.

There are few situations in which a psychiatrist or other mental health professional can break confidentiality. However, one such situation is when a therapist becomes aware of his or her patient's intention to kill someone else. The therapist is legally allowed to warn the intended victim and perhaps notify the local police. This allowance was generated by case law, specifically *Tarasoff v. the Regents of the University of California,* decided by the California Supreme Court, in which the UC Berkeley student counseling service was held liable when it did not break patient confidentiality to warn a potential murder victim of a stated threat to kill her. The 1976 case, sometimes called Tarasoff I, concluded that a therapist has a "duty to warn" an intended victim. The court "ruled that a physician or psychotherapist who has reason to believe that a patient may injure or kill someone must notify the potential victim."[4] Tarasoff II was decided by the California Supreme Court in 1982, and in it the "duty to warn" was broadened to include a "duty to protect" as well. By the early 1990s, the proper noun *Tarasoff* had become a verb. Your supervisor might ask, "And did you Tarasoff him?"[5]

Dealing with Tarasoff situations can be particularly stressful. First, you're dealing with a person who is capable of planning and committing a heinous act of violence. Second, preventing the death of a potential murder victim, someone who isn't even your own patient, is vitally important.

. . .

Believing honesty to be the best policy in this situation, I briefly tell Mr. Pauletti about Tarasoff and the attendant dilemmas that spring from those court decisions. He seems to listen with interest and understanding. So I plunge into the assessment, hoping blindly that he will cooperate.

"What's your boss's name?"

"Charlie Owens."

"Phone number? Address?"

He gives me the number. "You can ask for him. He's a supervisor over there. I don't know the exact address, but . . ."

"That's okay," I reply, dumbfounded but grateful at Mr. Pauletti's willingness to spill the beans. "Remember, you don't have to tell me everything if you don't want to, but I am asking you so I can help you. I just want you to know clearly that the law allows me to call him and warn him of your homicidal plans, and the police to come and interview you." I pause before asking the big question: "How are you planning to do it?"

Mr. Pauletti becomes downright animated as he explains his particular method of enacting murder. He has gone to the library, in these pre-Internet days, to check out books explaining how to make detonating devices and bombs that are difficult to detect. He wants to construct a bomb out of usual household materials and simple chemicals that can be ordered by catalog.

He tells me that he has already gathered ammonia, corn syrup, and industrial acids, which he is storing in a closet, under lock and key, at home. He plans to place the bomb under his boss's car. He goes on to tell me of his capacity to design an elaborate system of radio control so that he can detonate the bomb while observing his boss driving down the exit road from his warehouse. As he talks, Mr. Pauletti appears to be thoroughly enjoying himself. He then tells me about his prior experience with explosives.

"I was one of the technical guys of an artillery unit. We were pretty far behind the lines, and the war was in its later stages. I had a dangerous job. I would have been the second-to-last guy out if we would have had to bug out. I liked it. I thought it was a thrill. It was exciting to practice detonations with live ammo. But when they came to close our unit down, I felt betrayed. They transferred me, gave me a demotion, a desk job. I was pissed. I thought we had done a great job. So I decided to get revenge. One day, one of the generals came through camp, and he demanded a small honor guard with some vehicles in a parade. Well, I got some live ammo and shot down his big-ass banner. They couldn't figure out who did it. I was that methodical. I eventually admitted to it, and the MPs took me away. They tied me to a bed and shot me up with Thorazine. I talked to a shrink. Then they court-martialed me and sent me away to a psych hospital. I was diagnosed as manic-depressive and schizophrenic. I was locked up for nine months in Kentucky."

I am feeling much relieved at Mr. Pauletti's willingness to talk. But obviously I am also disturbed at his homicidal risk, with its attendant secrecy and his apparently blithe attitude toward killing. My mission is not nearly accomplished. "Have you thought about the consequences for yourself if you actually do kill your boss?"

"Of course," he says. "But this plan is so good I'll never get caught. And if, by chance, I do get caught and end up in jail, I'd waste no time in killing myself. I couldn't stand being in jail."

"But . . . the possibility of going to jail, where you would kill yourself, is not enough to prevent you from killing your boss?"

"Listen, doc," he says, his voice rising slightly, his face flushing a bit, "I told you that this plan is so airtight that nobody will be able to trace the ingredients of the bomb. I can easily make it look like an accident, like an exploding car engine and fire, stuff that happens often enough without a bomb going off. I can be deadly. I'm one of the most dangerous people I know." He stares at me coldly, then continues: "And since you're the only person other than me who knows about me wanting to kill my boss, the only way I'd get caught is if you told the authorities."

"Okay," I say tentatively.

"And I just may have to take out anyone else who knows about it." My patient, on our first visit, ostensibly an evaluation, fixes me with a cold, hard glare, his body remaining motionless.

Holy shit, I think. What gives here? This damn guy threatens to kill me and looks so calm about it. Now, bear in mind that psychiatrists are used to getting death threats. I have already been intimidated this way at least a half dozen times in my two-year career. The only difference is that all those threats came from extremely drunk or rabidly paranoid patients who either would not remember making the threat or could not muster the planning and organization skills it would take to actually hunt me down and dispose of me.

Invariably these threats would come when I informed patients of something they didn't want to hear, such as when I told a malingering patient, "Get the hell out of my ER! I don't believe for a second you are actually going to kill yourself," or told a manic hell-bent on being discharged, "Sorry, sir, but I am going to hospitalize you, because I feel you're making very poor decisions due to your mental illness." Maybe the libertarian psychiatrist Thomas Szasz was right, and we psychiatrists are, on our Kafkaesque common path, now merely tools of society, agents of behavioral and social control.

But the blast of menace emanating from Mr. Pauletti wakes me from this existential slumber. "And I just may have to take out anyone else who knows about it."

I look at him and nod slightly. He continues to stare, not particularly hostile, not particularly welcoming; he's defiant and expectant. I take a full thirty seconds to formulate my response. Mr. Pauletti says nothing more, perhaps realizing that, when a challenge has been thrown down, it is only fair to give the presumed opponent enough time to generate an answer, something like the slow countdown before pistols are drawn in a duel.

A lightbulb goes off in my head. Eureka! "The part of our brain that leaps to conclusions like this is called the adaptive unconscious," writes Gladwell. "The adaptive unconscious does an excellent job of sizing up the world, warning people of danger, setting goals, and initiating action in a sophisticated and efficient manner."[6]

Despite my excitement, I rein myself in and speak slowly, deliberately, evenly, so as to not telegraph my fear. Dogs can smell fear. Predators, too, can sense fear. They live for the smell of it. "I'll be honest, Mr. Pauletti, I feel threatened by what you just said. But, what I don't get is how you think I can help you if you come in here to get help from me and you're threatening me. I need to be intact and operating without intimidation if I can be of any help to you. I can't help you if you're threatening me." I appeal to his sense of self-preservation, if he indeed has any. "If you want me to help you," I say, "then you're going to have to take back that threat. If you can't do that, then I suggest that you leave now and go find someone else to help you." This was a big gamble.

I see that Sal Pauletti is left speechless by this remark. Inside, I am goddamned proud of myself. I believe what I say. It's the bald-faced truth. It's clear. It's nonthreatening. I find out later from at least one of my supervisors that it is about the best (and only) thing I could have said if I was going to have any chance of helping this patient. I then realize that my open-minded, seat-of-the-pants, stream-of-consciousness, living-in-the-moment interpersonal style, which will make me a good emergency psychiatrist, is a definite bonus in dealing in the here and now with a homicidal maniac. I find out that my instincts are good. I pass a test.

I might be in good company. According to a study of decision making among emergency first responders cited by Gladwell, "People who make decisions under pressure . . . don't logically and systematically compare all available options. That is the way people are taught to make decisions, but in real life it is much too slow. . . . Nurses and firefighters would size up a situation almost immediately and *act,* drawing on experience and intuition and a kind of rough mental simulation."[7]

The rest of the session goes well. Mr. Pauletti agrees to dispose of his bomb-making equipment and to come back and see me early the following week. He agrees to let me write a note to the manager at his workplace, requesting a medical leave of absence for treatment. Per confidentiality laws, I do not need to reveal Mr. Pauletti's condition or his treatment to his supervisor. He agrees to this leave from work, which will remove him from contact with his supervisor. He agrees to seek out group therapy for anger management.

I decide not to subject Mr. Pauletti to involuntary hospitalization as a "danger to others." And I take a calculated risk and decide not to Tarasoff his supervisor, because this would only alienate my patient. Mr. Pauletti, visibly much, much calmer, takes his leave from me and agrees to come at 11 A.M. on Monday for a second session. I bid him adieu and close my office door and slump into my chair, exhausted. I have ten minutes until my next appointment.

My next patient, Mrs. Watson, a self-diagnosed manic-depressive who insists on taking lithium, complains excessively to me about how bored she is with her husband. She goes through the same diatribe every week. I listen politely and stifle yawns while she goes on. No complaints here. She's not suicidal or homicidal and seems unable to muster an erotic transference, thank God. After she leaves, I have two more patients with straightforward problems.

It's five thirty, and I have paperwork to do. I feel a rising tide of anxiety about Mr. Pauletti. Did I let him off the hook too easily? Would I not see him again? Would he just go off and annihilate his supervisor despite his assurances to me that he would not? My gut told me that his willingness to discuss his homicidal thoughts and his willingness to take so many protective steps must have reduced the risk greatly. But I know I'm taking a chance on this one, and I decide I'd better check in with as many supervisors as I can in the next day or two and figure out if I'm on the right track. Still, my fledgling judgment tells me that my shaky therapeutic alliance with Mr. Pauletti would be just so much dust in the wind if I notify his supervisor of his homicidal thoughts and plans. I'm comforted by the fact that the fine print of an authoritative psychiatric textbook states, "The Tarasoff I ruling does not require therapists to report a patient's fantasies; instead it requires them to report an intended homicide, and it is the therapist's duty to exercise good judgment."[8]

. . .

I call the extension of my caseload supervisor nervously, wanting to let her know about this hot potato of a case and feeling that I need to get some perspective. She panics, which to me seems to reflect her own insecurities; it sounds like her mouth goes dry and her throat tightens. She grills me for details about the interview and mumbles something about needing to tell the director of the Outpatient Department about the case. I tell her I think that's a fine idea.

"Are you sure that's okay? I'll call you tonight," she concludes. I looked to her for guidance, but she has punted. Her anxiety fuels mine.

I decide to phone a previous supervisor, one who has been an attending physician on the inpatient psychiatric ward for more than ten years and who is developing a genuine expertise in forensic matters. Forensic psychiatry is a subspecialty that examines legal issues, both civil and criminal, as they apply to the practice of psychiatry. I trust her judgment, but I know she's from a strong biomedical psychiatric tradition and is fairly rigid and conservative in her management. And, subconsciously, I know she is going to scare the daylights out of me when I call her. She does not disappoint. She is absolutely horrified that I didn't give the patient's supervisor a Tarasoff warning. She doesn't exactly call me negligent, because she agrees that I did take measures to protect the intended victim, but, upon hearing the details of the case, she emphatically says that she would have placed the patient on an involuntary hold, admitted him to the inpatient psychiatric ward, called the police, called Mr. Pauletti's supervisor to warn him, and prescribed heavy sedatives.

Okey-dokey, I think. "Thank you very much," I say. "I am following up with my caseload supervisor and the director of the outpatient clinic."

That evening, as I drink beer and watch sitcoms with my wife, my caseload supervisor calls me. She essentially tells me that the Outpatient Department's director, a prominent psychoanalyst, thinks I did the right thing by not antagonizing the patient, by making him feel welcome to come back, by doing just enough to temporarily protect the intended victim, and by making the ultimate intervention—that of ensuring rapport between myself and the patient. As a result, he will come back and see me and engage in a psychotherapy that will only further reduce the risk that he will execute his supervisor.

So, from three different psychiatrists with three different levels of experience and three different areas of expertise, I get three different perspectives. One of the first bromides I heard— on my first rotation as a psychiatric resident—came from my young attending at San Francisco General Hospital: "The only thing that two psychiatrists can agree on is that a third one is wrong."

My former inpatient attending, the conservative forensic expert, later offered me this piece of wisdom (which seems to run counter to her cut-and-dried view of the world): "You can ask ten different psychiatrists what they might do in a given situation, and you might get ten different answers. And it's possible that none of them would be wrong."

Kaplan and Sadock weigh in on the question: "Since [Tarasoff,] courts and state legislatures have increasingly held psychiatrists to a fictional standard of having to predict the future behavior [dangerousness] of their potentially violent patients. Research has consistently demonstrated that psychiatrists cannot predict future violence with any dependable accuracy."[9]

This is a hard lesson, learned early in my career. The clinical uncertainty is frightening. I am discovering what I had already suspected. Psychiatrists are not much better than anybody else at predicting patients' behavior. And, when predicting whether an individual will act on suicidal or violent thoughts after discharge from a hospital or emergency room, psychiatrists can really anticipate only the next few hours of behavior.

According to Simon, "Assessing the risk of violence is a lot like weather forecasting: pretty good for the very immediate future and not so good for the longer term."[10] And they call economics the dismal science? Assessment has gotten a bit more scientific over the years, though, with the development of the Iterative Classification Tree, an actuarial method for violence risk assessment, by the MacArthur Foundation and numerous forensic psychologists and psychiatrists in 2000. Yet, probably for a variety of reasons—one being that it's a relatively cumbersome tool—it has been only rarely applied in the inpatient wards and psychiatric emergency rooms of the nation.[11]

. . .

Sal Pauletti returns for his appointment on Monday. He looks better, and he actually sits in his chair and talks to me in a lucid and calm manner. He still has issues, but his homicidality has dissipated, if not disappeared. I was relieved to discover that he had actually started a two-week break from work and that the sedative-tranquilizer medication that I had prescribed was already helping to reduce his irritability and insomnia. Mr. Pauletti had also disposed of his bomb-making materials.

"You know, last week, doc, when I was tapping the room all over? I was searching for a soft spot, a spot underneath the Sheetrock where there wasn't a stud. I was planning to pound in your walls, smash up your office. I didn't want to break my hand. So that's why I was checking the walls. When I was sitting in the waiting room, I was fully planning to trash your office."

"What stopped you?" I ask.

"I don't know what it was, but it was something about the way you handled me and handled yourself that I decided not to do it."

"Thank you," I say. Amen, I think.

His anger at his boss essentially disappeared when he removed himself from the workplace. I saw Mr. Pauletti several more times over the ensuing weeks, and, ultimately, he decided that he could afford an early retirement, planning to start a small business.

FOUR

THE PSYCHODYNAMO

Learning to Listen with a Professional Ear

For all its headaches, psychiatric training is made rich by one's interaction with supervisors. In looking for my own psychotherapy mentor, I searched for an approachable, practical, user-friendly psychiatrist—one whom, in an ideal world, I could model myself after.

The late Dr. David Viscott writes in his classic *The Making of a Psychiatrist,* "You can tell a bastard from a nice guy in a moment if you have any sense at all."[1] I knew I had discovered one of the good ones when I met my first psychotherapy supervisor, a psychiatrist named Chesley Herbert. Ches, who had already been in private practice for more than ten years, seemed to be a regular guy, and he made me feel comfortable during our meetings. I could identify with him.

Ches was not wedded to any particular theory. He had trained at San Francisco's Langley Porter Psychiatric Institute in the mid-to-late 1970s, an era when Freudian psychoanalytic theory held sway, but, given his personality, he was not well suited to the detached, aloof, omniscient psychoanalytic stance in vogue at the time. He likely crafted his own style of therapy, and while it was certainly informed by his theoretical training, he was not in lockstep with others in any particular philosophical framework.

The psychiatrists Thomas Lewis, Fari Amini, and Richard Lannon describe the matter of crafting a style in their fascinating book *A General Theory of Love:* "The *person* of the therapist is the converting catalyst, not his order or credo, not his spatial location in the room, not his exquisitely chosen words or denominational silences. . . . The dispensable trappings of dogma may determine what a therapist *thinks* he is doing, what he talks about when he talks about therapy, but the agent of change is who he *is*."[2]

And given his experience, Ches was in a position to gently indoctrinate me in my role as psychotherapist. We met at 7:45 A.M. on Tuesdays, as the rest of his schedule was filled.

At our first meeting, Ches was dressed in an unassuming navy sport jacket and gray slacks. He wore wire-rim glasses and had short brown hair cut almost military style. In my tiny basement office, he would sit across from me, his hands gently pressed together above his lap as he listened intently.

"But what do I have to offer someone in therapy?" I ask. "I've never done it before."

"Don't sell yourself short. You've already learned how to listen with a professional ear. You're intelligent. You're well trained. You have good intentions." He laughs at this. "You know what I mean."

"Yeah," I say.

"You're in this to be helpful. You're fresh. You're not burned out. You will be present in the room and listening carefully. What you actually say will not be all that important."

"What?" I ask incredulously.

"Well, let me rephrase that. It is important to be aware of what you say and how you say it, because you are trying to gauge the patient's reactions and to follow the narrative of the interaction. But there are many, many different ways to phrase questions and make comments, and few of them would be wrong things to say."

"I understand what you mean," I say. "So, my first visit with my first psychotherapy case is next week. How should I prepare?"

"Well, two things come to mind. First is, as you're listening, keep in the back of your head what makes a good psychotherapy candidate, and observe if he has these attributes or not."

"You mean the basics, like intelligence, insight, psychological-mindedness, motivation, ability to think abstractly?"

"Exactly. And is he someone who takes responsibility for his life, or is he someone who is always blaming other people? Is he willing to take responsibility for his thoughts, feelings, behaviors? That's a good sign."

"Okay, check," I say. "And what's the other thing?"

"I know this may seem silly, but, get a pen and paper, okay? I'm going to give you a handful of queries and questions that are good kindling material for a therapy evaluation if things start to flounder."

Ches helps me generate the following list, which seems like a list of questions from a blue-book examination or a job interview from hell:

Describe someone important in your life.

Describe one of the happiest, or best, moments of your life.

Describe one of the saddest, or worst, moments of your life.

Any recurrent dreams? What do you make of them?

How would you like to be? What would it feel like to be that way? What would be good about it? What would be bad about it?

Nearing the end of my hour of supervision, Ches asks me, "Any questions?"

Only about a million, I think. "Yes, but nothing pressing," I say. "I bet I'll have even more next week."

"I'm sure you'll do well," says Ches, "and, if your patient shows up, we'll have a lot to talk about."

"Thanks, Dr. Herbert, I appreciate your help."

. . .

The first two years of psychiatric residency are an indoctrination into the white-coated medical model of psychiatry. We are the doctors. You are the patient. Ours is a particularly mismatched relationship. You are *not* a person. You *are* a set of symptoms—along with physical signs and laboratory and radiological findings—that I am to diagnose via algorithmic logical thinking in order to find the ideal treatment for your malady. You will be the recipient—the beneficiary—of my medical wisdom.

Four years of medical school, a year of internship, then a year as a biomedical psychiatrist on the inpatient ward and the consultation-liaison service: all are set aside when you embark on the solitary path of becoming an in-the-office psychiatrist. Those six years of blood, sweat, and tears recede into the background of your day-to-day work life. A major obstacle to becoming a full-fledged psychiatrist, with knowledge of both the mind *and* the brain, is the integration of your identity as a "real" doctor with your emerging sense of self as a psychotherapist. I was both skeptical and anxious about this process. I am, by nature, well meaning, friendly, and somewhat psychologically minded. However, I did not feel old enough, or wise enough, to advise folks on how they should live their lives. Before I started my psychotherapy training, I suffered from a misconception of what it was all about. I thought it consisted of giving advice, instructing, and counseling people on what to do and how to do it.

Psychotherapy instruction in 1990 came delivered in an old package: the apprenticeship model of education. Psychotherapy research was then a field in its infancy. At the time, the practice of psychotherapy was not dictated or directed by an "evidence base" derived from clinical studies. Becoming a psychotherapist was a matter of learning by doing, although it involved more than simply flying by the seat of your pants: residents attended lectures on psychological principles for two to three hours a week. But we received no specific training in counseling technique, as one might in a graduate program of psychology. We just did it.

During our third-year seminars, we became steeped in psychodynamic theory, and not just in Freud. Other (generally clearer and more useful) theoreticians like Melanie Klein, George Winnicott, Heinz Kohut, and John Bowlby and their respective theories—on object relations, the experience of therapy as an "emotional container," self-psychology, and attachment theory—too were presented and discussed. At team meetings in the Outpatient Department, we formally presented our most psychologically charged cases and prepared extensive psychodynamic formulations. We also learned by presenting process notes in weekly meetings with psychotherapy supervisors, most of whom were experienced psychiatrists in private practice. These notes described the flow of a therapy session and allowed student and teacher to break down the psychodynamics in play during a given session.

Much of a resident's caseload, which totals about forty patients, is composed of "med management" patients with whom one does not do traditional psychotherapy. Many of these patients are chronically ill, but relatively stable on antipsychotic medications, mood stabilizers, antidepressants, or some combination of these. Some are higher-functioning patients who take antidepressants or antianxiety medications and receive their psychotherapy from psychologists or master's-level therapists. These folks are seen, at most, every two weeks, sometimes only once every two to three months, for fifteen- to thirty-minute sessions in which the focus is on medication compliance, benefits, and side effects.

My psychotherapy education began in earnest when I was a third-year resident. In 1990, the dawning of the "Decade of the Brain," I enlisted for what I would come to call psychotherapy boot camp. I would find myself bandied about in a titanic war between the last gasps of Freudian psychoanalysis, representing psychology, and the growing juggernaut of the neurosciences, representing biology. Political power within organized psychiatry at this time was polarized between Freudian psychoanalysts at one end and bench scientists at the other. Most clinical practitioners, and those of us in training, were stuck in the middle.

"Reductionism of either the biological or the psychological variety calls to mind the adage that if one's only tool is a hammer, everything can begin to look like a nail. Patients may be shortchanged by hard-nosed and inflexible diagnostic and therapeutic approaches that are reductionistic in either the biological or the psychological direction," writes Harvard psychiatrist David Brendel, author of *Healing Psychiatry*.[3] The influence of biomedical psychiatrists was definitely on the rise.

In fact, as I examine my "process notes" from those days, I see that many are jotted on the backs of biomedical papers—one bears a highly schematic rendering of the dopamine receptor; another is an article about the use of depot antipsychotic medications—preparations injected in the muscle and lasting up to four weeks—to treat cocaine dependence.

Lewis, Amini, and Lannon describe white-coated devotees of Science like this: "Neuroscientists understand the immediate chemical effect of a handful of medications, but connecting the dots of those minute molecules to sketch human actions, thoughts, feelings, and traits means tracing a baffling, blossoming tangle of biochemical events."[4] On dogmatic psychoanalysts, they have this to say: "Some therapists recoil from the pivotal power of relatedness. They have been told to deliver insight—a job description evocative of estate planning or financial consulting, the calm dispensation of data packets from the other side of an imposing desk."[5] How was I to reconcile my self-identity as an aggressive, devil-may-care cowboy psychiatrist with that of a seemingly passive, introspective, sensitive psychotherapist?

I would need to learn how to integrate information from both biology and psychology to become a capable clinical psychiatrist. Not surprisingly, this involves a process; it's not something that can be accomplished overnight. "Like the rest of medicine, psychiatry is a craft. . . . A young psychiatrist—skilled, competent, articulate—learns to *do* psychiatry, not so much to describe what she does. She learns her psychiatry the way a young violinist learns to play the violin. For someone who is good at her task, these ways of perceiving settle in so deeply that they become the way the person moves, hears, and observes when at that task," writes Luhrmann.[6]

.   .   .

Before seeing my first new patient, I review the notes of his four-visit outpatient evaluation, which were written by Dr. Nelson, a senior resident known for his thoroughness and intellectual capacity. I make an only superficial mental note of the biomedical diagnoses, drawn from the *Diagnostic and Statistical Manual of Mental Disorders* (DSM-III, the then-current third edition of the diagnostic guidelines published by the American Psychiatric Association): Dysthymic Disorder and/or Major Depressive Disorder, recurrent, moderate and/or Social Phobia on Axis I and a rule-out of Obsessive-Compulsive Personality Disorder on Axis II. Dysthymic disorder refers to chronic low-grade depression, often dating back to childhood. Axis I is where the major psychiatric disorders are coded. Axis II is available to code for the presence of a personality disorder. These are part of the DSM's system for constructing a set of psychiatric diagnoses for a particular patient. What can these labels really tell you about an individual? They are only marginally helpful to a psychiatrist looking to embark on a course of psychotherapy. They provide only blurry, rough boundaries that mark the individual as being prone to depression, anxiety, shyness, and obsessive thinking.

Before that first visit, I experience a keen case of performance anxiety. Would I do it right? Is there a "right" way to commence psychotherapy? What are the best ways? What major gaffes might I commit? Would I have the necessary patience for the visit? Would I get bored? Would I know what to say, how to say it, when to say it? Should I just look wise, scratch my chin, and look thoughtful?

I go out to the modest waiting room at one o'clock on the dot. "Are you Mr. Wolf?"

The man sitting in the chair looks up, clears his throat, and says, "Yes."

I introduce myself, and he stands up and offers his right hand to me. "Nice to meet you. I'm Jared Wolf."

Instinctively I shake his hand, though devout Freudians would have discouraged that social nicety, contaminating, as it might, the opening moments of an emerging transference.

Viscott economically describes transference in *The Making of a Psychiatrist:* "Therapy often seems . . . (silly or farfetched) . . . to those who have no personal experience with it. . . . But the patient's feelings about his doctor often reflect how he feels about important people in his family as well as the doctor. The feelings are real but to the outsider they seem out of place. They *are;* they're transferred."[7]

I can feel already that it will be difficult for me to maintain a detached psychoanalytic stance, to be the second coming of Freud. I will have to make do with common sense and gut instincts in working with my first bona fide psychotherapy candidate, and sort it out later in supervision.

"Pleased to meet you as well," I say quietly. "Come this way. My office is just down the hall."

"Thank you," he says.

Tall, with a receding hairline, thin except for a slight pot-belly, casually dressed in blue jeans and a plaid long-sleeve shirt,

Mr. Wolf, looking a tad anxious, sits down in a slightly padded straight-backed chair across from me. My chair, which is identical, stands about four feet away. At my neophyte level of training, I have neither a fancy Eames recliner nor a psychoanalytic couch.

With cheat sheet and clipboard in hand, I feel prepared. But before I say a word, Mr. Wolf speaks, registering a minor complaint about the billing system in place at Langley Porter at the time. Such housekeeping details—regarding billing, duration of sessions, cancellation policies, and so on—generally are addressed at the start of a session. All but the strictest Freudians address these matters up front. Talking about money and the meaning of money—who is taking care of whom in the relationship?—is an important aspect of the opening stages of psychotherapy. It can get confusing when one is a trainee, because the bills go directly from the institution to the patient, and the checks go straight from patient to institution. Though a few of my supervisors strongly encourage me to have my patients pay me directly (with a check written out to the institution), I never do get into this habit. In my family and hometown culture, it was not polite to talk about money. Moreover, I feel I don't deserve to charge the patient anything for my time because I am a novice—a good example of my own neurotic self-devaluing, a sort of pseudohumility.

"Is it okay if I take notes while we talk?" I ask.

"By all means," Mr. Wolf answers.

"Where should we begin?" I ask.

"How much of the evaluation did you see?"

"I reviewed all of it. I spoke with Dr. Nelson about it as well. But I would like to hear your story from you. What's uppermost in your mind?"

Mr. Wolf begins by succinctly and articulately summarizing his concerns: a dead-end career, years of severe depression, shyness, self-loathing, anger turned inward, a lack of initiative, and a feeling of stagnation and hopelessness. "I've been going through this for years and years. I finally got sick of it," he says, "so I decided to come in here."

Bravo! I think. A strong opening! He demonstrates to me the virtues of self-knowledge, clarity, and motivation. Amazingly enough, as I look over my process notes years later, these were among the most important issues we dealt with over the course of three years of psychotherapy, most of it once a week but some of it twice a week.

"It takes a lot of courage to look at your issues," I say. "I'm glad you came in." Oops, should I have said that last thing? Do I need him to take care of my needs? I take a deep breath. Just be yourself, I tell my Self. Sometimes a cigar is just a cigar.

"The fact that I'm here . . ." His voice trails off. "I don't know how severe it is." His face becomes tight, and he reels himself back in. He becomes silent and looks stricken.

Should I say, "Yeah, dude, you seem pretty messed up to me?" Or, "Nah, don't worry about it?" Obviously these are wrong responses. Since the truth rests somewhere in the middle, I remain quiet. Not knowing exactly what to say in the moment, I retreat to my cheat sheet. Soon enough I would learn to "follow the affect," meaning to consistently observe a patient's visible expressions of emotion and to correlate them with the content of what he or she is saying. This time-honored piece of supervision helps keep the therapist on track.

"For me to get to know you better, tell me what was the best time in your life."

He seems to relax with the question and pauses briefly. "There's never been a time when things have gone perfectly," he says. "Things have gone very well at times—when I've been in a great relationship, when my writing is going well, when I've completed a very difficult task, when I've been recognized by my peers."

"Why is recognition so satisfying?" Follow the path, take what the patient gives you.

"It happens so rarely. I have a pattern of connecting my self-worth to what others think of me. I'm now trying to get that feeling from within. Trying to believe in myself."

His face brightens a bit, and I think, "Bingo!" Here's a guy who is willing to take responsibility for his own feelings and mature enough to seek help, to try to get better. And what are we—maybe ten minutes into this thing?

He then gets excited telling me about his ideas for writing a novel. But shortly afterward he becomes downcast, reminded somehow of his proclivity for procrastination.

"Well, that's one of the reasons you came in," I say earnestly. "We can look at that."

He again becomes befuddled, talking abstractly about "looking at variables," about recognizing patterns and rhythms and syncopations, about finding order. Trying desperately to apply logic to an emotionally twisted situation. As he runs from his feelings and retreats into his intellect, he appears ever more fretful and sad. It is as if he is trying to insulate himself from feeling too good, too confident, too expansive.

Ah, the wonderful self-destructive thoughts of depression, I think. I must gently usher him back into the wider expanses of other emotions. "You mentioned being 'in a great relationship.' What made it great?" I ask.

"Well, I had an eight-month relationship end a few years ago. We had companionship and intimacy—finishing each other's sentences, knowing each other nonverbally, cooking together, leaving little messages for each other, being physically side by side, great sex."

"How were you feeling at the time?"

"Whole."

We spend much of the rest of the session dissecting the relationship and the breakup. What went well? What could have been done better? What were the points of tension? What, if anything, could have prevented the breakup?

We end the session talking about Mr. Wolf's unexpected success in tennis in high school. He came to the game late and went on to place in the finals at state. He described the elation he felt at achieving athletically. Despite all that, he was frequently teased at school for being "nerdy." He mentioned having several "closet friends" who did things with him discreetly after school, but who joined many others in heaping scorn on him during the school day. Now, in retrospect, he could see that he had played a submissive role in those relationships, and the passivity, experiencing it again now, almost fifteen years later, feels intolerable.

I finish with a summary statement of sorts: "I'm glad you came in. I think we can work together to look at issues. I appreciate your candor and honesty and openness. I think we can look at ways to help you operate better in the world."

"Thanks. It got to the point where I had to do something," he says.

We set the second appointment for next week—same day, same time. Providing consistency is important to beginning and sustaining a therapy. Or so I am told.

. . .

After Mr. Wolf leaves, I breathe a sigh of relief. I give myself a B plus. And I am a little bit excited. It seems like he is a good candidate for psychotherapy.

Rather than anticipating that I would reconstruct the session from memory, I chose to take notes along the way. I knew from working as a journalist in the past that I would have a difficult time re-creating much of the conversation from memory alone. And, as in journalism, I was looking for quotes that would somehow summarize a feeling, a state of mind. The disadvantage of this method is that it constructs a barrier between you and your patient. It can be distracting. It may make the patient feel a bit like a specimen. But the advantage is that the patient knows you have a better chance of internalizing his comments; and, in fact, it allows you to go back over the notes later.

Process notes can be used to draw a tentative map of a person's psychology. In constructing this map you strive to capture the unique qualities and interrelationships between the patient's different psychological attributes. The greatest advantage for me is that the clipboard, paper, and pen give me something to do, keep my hands busy and my eyes occupied, and allay my anxiety, which could easily manifest itself in the form of restless hands, eyes, or feet during the session.

As I look over my chicken-scratched notes, I have an opportunity to ask myself a lot of tough questions:

What was the patient's affect (meaning facial expression), especially in relation to the content of the discussion?
What caused his affect or his thought content to shift?
What did his body language indicate?

What sorts of questions brought out the most authentic and important information?

What was most important in what he said?

How can I learn to listen for what's most important?

How did his behavior match already known patterns of psychological defenses, issues, and diagnoses?

What, if any, themes emerged over the course of a session?

When was he avoiding potentially emotionally charged subjects?

Did it matter what I said? How I asked questions? If I made summary or supportive or other types of statements?

When I meet with Ches the following week, I give him a standard medical-student/psychiatric-resident presentation on Mr. Wolf: "Mr. Jared Wolf is a thirty-four-year-old never married, Caucasian, nonpracticing Christian gentleman with no formal psychiatric history who referred himself for psychotherapy via Langley Porter's OPD [Outpatient Department] Intake Clinic. He was diagnosed as having probable Social Phobia, Dysthymic Disorder with a rule-out of current Major Depression, and a rule-out of Obsessive-Compulsive Personality Disorder. He has no active medical problems. He has a negative history of psychiatric admissions, suicide attempts, violence, or even suicidal ideation. This is his first time in outpatient psychiatric treatment." Et cetera, et cetera, et cetera. You get the idea.

This kind of presentation—a practical shorthand familiar to all physicians—contains the kind of information that is gathered in a biomedical model type of psychiatric evaluation. It allows student and mentor to share a basic understanding of a patient. It stands in stark contrast to a psychodynamic formulation, the presentation of which can go on for hours and includes copious details and examples of a patient's developmental history, the nature of his relationships, his most commonly used defense mechanisms, and the sources of tension, anxiety, or conflict in his life.

The presentation and discussion of a psychodynamic assessment are not nearly as telegraphic and are not communicated in shorthand. More accurately, they are an abridged version of a person's emotional life and work best in a narrative format, documenting not only the elements of a person's life story but also the arc of his psychological development. I hadn't yet learned how to identify all such details and how to deliver that kind of presentation, but I at least knew the type of information a psychotherapist-in-training was supposed to look for.

Without much fanfare, I review my process notes with Ches, sprinkling in recollections spurred by my review of the notes. Ches listens patiently as I laboriously present my process notes, a task that takes me ten to fifteen minutes.

"Good job. Certainly a fair amount of material here."

I'm not entirely sure what to make of that, so I nod my head tentatively.

"What kind of feeling did he generate in you?"

"Well," I start cautiously. "Mostly compassion. I could identify with his feelings of frustration and sadness, feelings I know I've had in the past."

"Okay, anything else?"

"I felt a little impatient at times and a little bored at others. It's hard to explain."

"Fair enough. As you know, your own response to a patient in the moment is referred to as countertransference. It can be a powerful tool for understanding an individual. I suggest you continue to pay attention to those feelings and note them, when you can, in your process notes, and we can talk about them."

Ches offers this advice in a straightforward manner, and it feels okay. It does not feel like he's trying to pry into my head space, which I'll admit was something I'd feared on the front end of this whole psychotherapy supervision thing. That sort of prying could make any good Midwesterner (you can take the boy out of Minnesota, but you can't take the Minnesota out of the boy) feel somewhat squeamish. The low-key, matter-of-fact way Ches does it makes a difference.

And this I know about myself: More than the average person, I respond to people according to how I'm feeling at the moment. I take my cues from my own response. It's partly an intuitive process, and it's definitely what one would call a gut process. I am what Jung called an "extroverted feeling" type, not the sort to become a Freudian psychoanalyst. Such a person would be my polar opposite—the mythical "introverted thinking" type.

"Okay, I'm sure I can do that," I tell Ches. "I stay pretty aware of my feelings on a moment-to-moment basis. Isn't it what psychiatrists are supposed to do?"

"Well," Ches says with a laugh, "not all of them know how. Although residency is four years, learning how to become a good psychiatrist can take a lifetime."

"I can believe it."

"So, back to the patient. I would say that Mr. Wolf has demonstrated a fair amount of courage and self-awareness in laying out just what it is he would like to accomplish in therapy. It's actually pretty impressive."

"I agree. He seemed very genuine to me as he talked."

"It's notable that he's so conflicted about his anger, and that feeling so confident in the moment makes him feel so anxious. You might want to look for him to withdraw, to become passive again at times, because it is in some ways a comfort zone for him. It may be that the patient will act passively with you here in the early going, and this may force you to be more active in asking questions. I would look for that to transpire over the next few sessions."

I think to myself, Now how in heck can he tell that from what I'd presented to him?

And then he bestows a supervisorial gem: "It's not logical," he says. "It's psychological."

"Oh," I say. "I like that one. What does it mean?"

"Mr. Wolf, due to his high intelligence and his tending toward avoidance and obsessive thinking, probably prefers to look at things logically. He is not as adept at looking at things in the context of feelings. He needs to develop his emotional intelligence, so to speak. So, you can tell him when he's trying to sort things out entirely with his left brain: 'It's not logical. It's psychological.'" My supervisor, with more than ten years of experience in a private, nearly full-time psychotherapy practice, is seemingly clairvoyant.

. . .

During the next two sessions, Mr. Wolf spends an inordinate amount of time talking about his progress in typing class. A typing class, for chrissakes! The guy is a real writer, one who

frequently jots down ideas on a notepad and is once again log-
ging several hours of writing time a week, and he refers to his
writing as "typing." He genuinely believes that the faster he
types, the better he writes. I also learn that he has been making
time graphs to analyze his efficiency.

Don't get me wrong. These are not bad ideas—taking typing
classes or trying to increase efficiency. But as my supervisor has
noted, these are attempts to mend a life via logic rather than via
emotional healing. Trying, trying, trying. Putting in a great
effort. Keeping things on a logical and superficial level to avoid
reaching deep emotions.

Over the next several weeks, I become more and more adept
at observing Mr. Wolf's body language and facial expressions,
especially as they change in response to the topic at hand. They
are usually congruent. At times I see him anxious or subdued;
at other times I see him confused, near-stuttering, and bewildered. But I also observe him smiling and confident and
relieved. I can feel myself becoming more sophisticated at
observing nonverbal behavior in a way that transcends the
medical model mental-status examination. So this is what it
feels like to discover the "stone tools" of psychotherapy. Hey, it
doesn't feel half bad.

. . .

An unfortunate by-product of this crash course in psychodynamic theory was that my fellow residents and I began to spend
an inordinate amount of time psychoanalyzing each other. We
pointed out others' defense mechanisms and alleged resistance
and traded stories of negative countertransference, because it
was fun and we needed the practice. Psychoanalytic principles

still dominated psychotherapy training at Langley Porter Psychiatric Institute in 1990.

By midyear many of my fellow residents had already commenced with their therapy cases. A number of my colleagues felt exhilarated by the prospect of learning to become psychotherapists. They were getting their patients up to twice-a-week sessions and seemingly effortlessly addressing such knotty issues as punctuality, missed appointments, and prompt payment of bills, and generally creating a system of rules for therapist and patient to live by. They had gone into psychiatry to become skilled psychotherapists who could dive right into an office practice after a four-year residency.

Or so I imagined. I, however, embraced my feelings of incompetence and inadequacy and pretended I didn't know much. I wasn't going to just throw away my personality and become a caricature of Freud. A few of my peers were so excited and felt so comfortable in the role of aloof therapist that they became almost smug, especially the ones channeling Freud, who generally prescribed a psychotherapeutic stance referred to as abstinence. To them I wanted to say, "Look, you're twenty-nine years old, you haven't finished your residency, you're not married, you don't have kids, you don't have a mortgage, you don't even have a real job yet. What makes you the second coming of Freud?" But of course I didn't.

I did my best to learn the stance of a psychodynamic psychotherapist and see the utility in the neutral, blank-slate approach. As you can probably surmise, I had to work very hard to develop this stance. Another of my mentors, Dr. Bob Buckley, who experienced the same difficulty, describes it well: "I have all of these painful memories of residency: of doing therapy and just sitting there knowing all the things I'm not supposed to do. And feeling completely flummoxed about what I should do. Feeling like an utter fool. And having the patient think I'm an utter fool. And I hated it. I feel like I had to pass through that, with all those restrictions, in order to come out the other side and be able to use that stuff."

. . .

As I rifle through my stack of process notes almost twenty years later, I randomly start reading from a session about a year into psychotherapy with Mr. Wolf. We had been meeting twice a week for many months, and I had started him on Prozac, a low dose, ten milligrams a day, which had helped lift his depression and alleviate his shyness. I could witness a slow and steady metamorphosis before my very eyes.

At this particular session, he starts before I say anything other than hello. "I may have accidentally broken the drought. I was walking down the street, and the skies were very overcast and cloudy. I then said, 'I just wish the weather would definitively decide what to do.' And a minute later, it started pouring and I got drenched. That's probably the first time I've used the word *definitively* in five years. It's been a serious week for omens and coincidences. I've had some pretty strange dreams this week."

I remain silent as Mr. Wolf continues: "I see each of these dreams as the last scenes of movies, all of which involve the same thing—me doing simple but spectacular things that I've never done before. In the first, I am with a group of detectives who are looking at a lineup of criminals, and I am the guy who picks the criminal out.

"Another dream was a remake of the film *The Man Who Knew Too Much*. In this dream sequence, I grab a sniper's rifle and pick off a guy about a half-mile away. He's the bad guy who's about to kill my daughter. In the original movie it's the wife who nails the assassin to save her son."

He's getting in touch with his anger, using it for good purposes—rescuing someone who's innocent. The fact that his unconscious mind has substituted himself for the powerful mother as a rescuing force is remarkable because, in real life, Mr. Wolf's mother is an imposing figure. In fact, as an award-winning journalist, she is, in some ways, larger than life. The fact that he can identify with her and be just as powerful is truly noteworthy. I realize at the time that there is much to mine in the session, but I continue to say nothing.

"In another dream, I strap on a pair of skates for the very first time and get a perfect string of sixes in a figure skating competition. The dreams are simple to describe, but they all have me doing things that are almost impossible to pull off, and in the dreams I've done them just like that. The dreams are all neat and simple."

As an inexperienced therapist, I do not entirely realize the import of the dreams at the moment. But I find you can never go wrong if you are guided by the principle of curiosity rather than cure, and follow the patient's story with open-ended queries. I ask, "What else might the dreams have in common?"

He says, "They all involved highly competitive things, in fact two of them were life-and-death situations. They all involve things that I've never done before in real life. In the one, the police sniper says there's no way I can make the shot, but I grab the rifle and do it anyway.

"I know I had a wild one this morning because I woke up ungodly early. I've been waking up exhausted, like I've just run twenty miles. Or I wake up with a sore back. It feels like some huge internal thunderstorm has been going on."

I tell him, "What's odd is that the message in the dreams is so positive. What do you make of that contrast?"

He does not hesitate: "I can't help but wonder about the future. I was thinking about last week, when I figured out that all those knee-jerk negative reactions I was having were more often than not lies about myself. I'm orienting myself to the belief that fears I've had about my future are also lies. I am trying to deliberately steer myself in that direction. It's a matter of conscious decision-making."

I ask, "How might your recent dreams connect with that process?"

"I would say . . . the dreams are a contradiction or a refutation of the negative things I've always told myself about myself. I can give you a simple example. There's this saying: 'A good way to break into the film industry is with a well-written mystery.' I look at my stuff and I know I've got a pretty good manuscript— a start on three pretty good novels, in fact. With a few more rewrites, I think they'll be extremely good. Ninety-five percent of the mysteries out there are garbage, but I know these three are already among the other 5 percent, so I can play by a different set of rules. In fact I can choose to play by a set of rules that favors me."

"How would your rules be different?"

"Given that I think these manuscripts are as good as they are, people would be coming to me once the word got out. I'd be . . ." He closes his eyes and thinks intently. "I'd be in a better position to dictate the course of events. If I do enough work on my novels, they'll do the work for me."

"How does it feel to say that here?"

"It comes out really awkward for me because I don't have a history. I can say positive things, and I know them to be true, but the accompanying emotion is one of discomfort. I can't quite believe what I'm saying. It's sort of like these shoes, only a few days old. At first they were uncomfortable, but now they're broken in. It's not just a whole new way of talking about myself, but also a whole new way of feeling about myself. I basically need to break those feelings in.

"There's kind of an internal conflict. The old ways are not quite ready to pack up and leave—especially the emotions. The cautious side of me says, 'Nothing is ever that easy.' The cautious side of me is Murphy's Law. But I can tell you—the old ways don't feel too comfortable either."

I take a cautious stab at a mini-interpretation: "I would venture to say that the dreams you described today reflect this conflict. You feel confident, but that is countered by fatigue, by aches and pains."

He pauses before responding. "It feels like a reassurance that things are going to be a lot easier than they look." He stops again, and then stretches his arms upward and cracks his knuckles. "It feels like I'm just starting to wake up—in a psychological sense, too.

"I felt real groggy throughout this morning. I must have been groggy, because I didn't realize until I got here that I had packed my conflicts so far away. This feels like a new morning. I also feel like I need a cup of coffee on a metaphysical level. I am waking up from an old set of beliefs and ways of thinking.

I can't describe how strange it feels to talk about myself in positive terms. It feels like my internal organs are rearranging themselves. I have a tingling feeling in my arms. I'm not used to it. I'm waiting for myself to get thrilled and pleased and excited about it. But it's as if something inside of me is holding me back."

I ask, "What would be holding you back?"

"The old ways, the knee-jerk negativity, fears, timidity, my natural tendency to caution, which I usually like, but which is inappropriate in this situation. It's as if the new emotions have not settled into place. . . . It's kind of an uncomfortable feeling. . . . I kind of have this notion that things are a bit fragile."

"It sounds like your cautious side is trying to rein you in," I say.

"Well, as they say, 'Forewarned is forearmed.' The next few months will be really critical to whether I continue to make progress or have to start all over."

"No, you may lose a few steps here and there, but you won't have to start over. No way," I say firmly.

"Well, inaction now would make for a huge reversal. I have to try and make these feelings fit. I have to modify them until they fit. It kind of feels like housecleaning."

And then, doing what a psychotherapist-in-training must do from time to time, I examine the transference, just as we're getting to the last few minutes of the session. This is much like Viscott explains it. I hate drawing attention to myself, and I dislike the seeming artificiality of examining the transference, but, what the heck, I'll give it a shot.

"What are your feelings toward me right now, after having the conversation that we just had?"

"I appreciate the feedback," he says. "Sometimes even the misses clarify a situation enough so that it leads to a better understanding indirectly. I appreciate the effort. Even if the basic ideas don't work exactly, they still do on a certain level. It's an experience I felt a lot in graduate school. The advice was rarely so totally off that I had to ignore it."

"Fair enough, Mr. Wolf. I'm afraid our time is up for today. We can pick this up on Monday."

Before I could pat myself on the back for being such a precise interpreter and master therapist, his blunt appraisal adjusted my perspective. He was telling me something like: "Well, we're off to a pretty good start, but I could certainly fall back, and by the way, don't think you're such hot shit or that you're smarter than me. I still have a lot to teach you."

Three steps forward, two steps back.

. . .

I was finding that integrating the biomedical model and the psychotherapeutic model would not be easy. Luhrmann describes the dilemma this way: "Young psychiatrists are supposed to learn to be equally good at talk therapy and drug therapy, psychotherapy and biomedical psychiatry, and the American Psychiatric Association thinks that this integration is what training programs in psychiatry teach. . . . Yet they are taught as different tools, based on different models, and used for different purposes. Some psychiatrists do integrate them to some extent."[8]

You can count Peter Kramer as one who has pulled it off. Prozac had made its debut a few years before I began performing psychological calisthenics in psychotherapy boot camp, but Kramer's book *Listening to Prozac* had not yet been published. In it, he illuminates, clarifies, and attempts to bridge what's become a yawning chasm between pharmacology and psychology:

> Spending time with patients who responded to Prozac had transformed my views about what makes people the way they are. I had come to see inborn, biologically determined temperament where before I had seen slowly acquired, history-laden character. . . .
>
> Pharmacotherapy, when looked at closely, will appear to be as arbitrary—as much an art, not least in the derogatory sense of being impressionistic where ideally it should be objective—as psychotherapy. Like any other serious assessment of human emotional life, pharmacotherapy properly rests on fallible attempts at intimate understanding of another person. . . .
>
> I found it astonishing that a pill could do in a matter of days what psychiatrists hope, and often fail, to accomplish by other means over a course of years: to restore to a person robbed of it in childhood the capacity to play. . . .
>
> Listening to medication implies a crossing of boundaries, a mixing of categories—approaching pharmacology with the tools of the psychotherapist. And the therapist's posture is speculative and doubting. . . . Faced with the unique patient, the doctor brings to bear every talent, every memory, every inspiration he can call upon, without suffering limitation by discipline, convention, or the strict requirements of scientific proof. Or rather, the doctor oscillates between perspectives, the eclectic and the conventional. I believe that the notion of "criteria" for the guild needs, like other grand categories, to be both stated and undermined.[9]

With the help of people like Jared Wolf, Chesley Herbert, and dozens of other patients and supervisors, I learned what I could during my year in psychotherapy boot camp. I learned how to "do" psychotherapy and "be" a psychotherapist. I do feel as if I'm more than capable of integrating my psychodynamics and psychotherapy experiences into a better understanding of my patients in the psych ER.

Here is what I learned in brief. Ten pearls of psychotherapy (in no particular order):

Be present.

Create a safe environment.

Help the patient discover his or her own tools of self-examination.

Provide an emotional container.

It's not logical. It's psychological.

Reveal things about yourself only if doing so will help the patient. Don't do it to meet your own needs.

Follow the affect.

Take the middle path—do not be overly gratifying and solicitous, or overly detached and aloof.

It's okay to make errors of the head, but not errors of the heart.

Go where the patient leads you.

FIVE

THE JAILER

If You Want to Go, You Have to Stay

They are not the most violent patients. Neither are they the flashiest or the loudest. But they certainly are the smelliest. These are the patients carted against their will into psych emergency grumbling and muttering, preferring a dingy alley to the bright lights of the hospital. These are the ones you might see zonked out on the sidewalk, the ones you need to step over and around if you are to successfully navigate certain neighborhoods in San Francisco.

These are not the guys who aggressively "spare-change" you. No, these individuals are the ones who quietly sit in front of their hand-painted placards saying, "I won't lie, it's for beer," or are passed out. These folks are not usually suicidal or homicidal. But, you might ask, are they gravely disabled? Oh, yeah, definitely.

These are the people who receive homeless-outreach services, whether they want them or not. These are the folks who sometimes get pushed along when the police do a sweep. What do these guys want? Mostly they want to be left alone. But do they have a right to be left alone? "The way I think about this problem is in these terms: Do I want to defend their right to be free?

Or do I want to protect them?" explains my mentor, Dr. Bob Buckley.

I noted earlier that California's Welfare and Institutions Code section 5150 provides for the involuntary detainment of an individual for up to seventy-two hours, so that the person can undergo psychiatric evaluation to determine whether he or she is a danger to self or others or is gravely disabled. The layperson can easily understand the concept of being suicidal or homicidal. But gravely disabled? Technically it means that a person is unable to provide food, clothing, and shelter for himself or herself *because of a psychiatric illness.* The finding relies on a two-part equation—first, that one is unable to supply one's own basic needs, and, second, that this self-neglect can be directly attributed to the symptoms of a major psychiatric illness.

. . .

Ray Shellam is ushered through a double set of locked doors by two female police officers. He looks tired; his face is a blank, at least what can be seen of it behind a beard so large that a bird could nest in it. Mr. Shellam's odor, pretty much average compared to that of other chronic street dwellers I've encountered, comes with him. This includes the distinctly stinky smell of "street feet" and the aldehyde-rich scent of old, partially metabolized alcohol. Mr. Shellam looks (and smells) like a malt-liquor-and-chronic-psychosis kind of guy to me.

In general, the smells emanating from the most severely compromised homeless people derive from some combination of the following: feces, urine (both old and fresh), alcohol (old or fresh, depending), sweat, and greasy dirt (similar to the kind retrieved from underneath a mechanic's fingernails after a long day at work). The actual chemical involved in the latter two situations is something called 2-nonenal.[1]

Your olfactory lobe, hidden just beneath the thinnest part of the skull, the cribriform plate, can be found straight up your nose. This part of the brain, in close proximity to the outside world and to your brain's centers of memory and emotion, lights up like a Christmas tree in the presence of patients like this one.

"Any trouble bringing him in, officer?" asks Brian, the day's triage nurse.

"No, gentle as a lamb. No ID, not saying much. But his name and date of birth check out on the computer." Ray Shellam appears to be in his late fifties or early sixties, so I am surprised to learn that he is only forty-three years old. Living hard takes its toll, indeed. "I wasn't going to bring him in. You know, we've seen him for years. He sleeps in a little alley downtown. Never bothers anyone, maybe does a little spare-changin' for his beer. But there's a new owner of the camera shop on the corner, and he keeps calling 911 to move him along."

Until recently, the city seemed not to care too much about a person as long as he didn't harass or assault anyone, didn't have others calling 911 about him or her too often, and didn't collect too many tickets for "quality of life" nuisance crimes such as trespassing, public intoxication, disorderly conduct, misdemeanor assault, and drug intoxication or possession.

When Mayor Gavin Newsom of San Francisco announced his "Care Not Cash" plan, which was approved by the voters as Proposition N in 2002, and which substituted vouchers for housing and services in place of cash welfare payments, he also rolled out enhanced services for the homeless. One of his creations was the Homeless Outreach Team (the HOT team). The primary

goal of the HOT team, headed by Captain Niels Tangherlini of
the city's fire department, is to get the city's highest utilizers of
911 services off the streets—anywhere off the streets, be it jail or
the hospital or a long-term psychiatric lockup.

"What's that merchant expect, setting up shop on the edge of
the Tenderloin?" I ask the officers. One of San Francisco's most
impoverished neighborhoods, the Tenderloin, a.k.a. the TL, has
a high crime rate and is full of cheap hotels, streetwalking sex
workers, and drug dealers. The cops simply shrug their shoulders. They remove Mr. Shellam's handcuffs, and one of them
fills out the 5150 paperwork that justifies their bringing him to
San Francisco General Hospital for a psychiatric evaluation. (It
is SFPD policy to place 5150'd individuals in handcuffs to prevent AWOLs. On more than one occasion, someone has escaped
from 5150 detention and committed suicide.)

Mr. Shellam stands silently by the desk, saying nothing and
looking blankly at the triage nurse as Brian asks him questions.
An odoriferous aura surrounds him. "Mr. Shellam, do you have
any medical problems we need to know about?" asks Brian. Mr.
Shellam says nothing, seemingly lost in space.

I look over Brian's shoulder at the MHS-140, a city-generated
form that roughly tracks a patient's pattern of visits within the
San Francisco County mental health system. "Got a red chart?"
I ask, referring to a set of "shadow charts" that we keep—copies
of the latest psych emergency records—since we rarely get our
hands on the patient's true San Francisco General Hospital
records.

"Negative," says Brian. "Per the records, his case is not open
anywhere. Last seen here in 2002, a couple times in 1996; diagnosed schizophrenic both times. Was open briefly at South of

Market in 1996, but his case was closed right away. Must have stopped showing up."

"I wonder if he's been in prison or jail or out of town during those gaps?" I ponder aloud.

"Got no rap sheet from us other than tickets for vagrancy from a long time ago," says one of the officers.

"How long you lived in San Francisco?" asks Brian.

Mr. Shellam shifts from foot to foot, saying nothing until a slight spark of recognition shows in his milky blue eyes. "Fifteen years," he mumbles, his voice sounding as if he's swallowed broken glass.

"Hey, let's go into this room here and get you out of those clothes and into the shower. When did you last take a shower?" asks Brian.

"What month is it?"

"What month do you think it is?"

"Well, it's April, middle of the month or so," replies Mr. Shellam. "I don't know, the sixteenth?"

"Not bad. It's April eighteenth."

"So it bein' April and all, I probably had a shower late February, early March. Around Ash Wednesday, I think. I got the shower at church. Other than Christmas, it's the only day of the year I go to church."

"Whew," I say, pinching my nose shut, breathing through my mouth, as Brian strips off layer after layer of moist, dirt-caked clothes—three pairs of jeans, three shirts, a jacket, and an overcoat. The layers of damp and dirty sweat socks are the worst. As Brian peels off the last one, encrusted cotton wisps cling to dirty crevices on the soles of the patient's feet. Shellam winces as Brian whisks them off.

More than 250,000 sweat glands grace the foot. When moisture has no place to go, then the resident bacteria grow like wildfire, and their waste products, laced with the aforementioned 2-nonenal, have nowhere to hide. Voilà, industrial-strength stench-foot.

I used to joke about wishing I had a hospital-issued clothespin to snap over my nose when unseemly smells like this take over psych emergency. These days, I frequently breathe through my mouth or my shirtsleeve to avoid inhaling those lovely packets of chemicals. Sometimes I use a scratchy hospital towel as a bandana across my nostrils. The smells have gotten me to thinking about creating a machine to record and quantify smells. I don't have much mad scientist in me, but that's one project I do fantasize about.

"Whaddya say about taking a shower, Ray?" asks Brian. "Afterward, we'll get you some lotion for those feet. They sure look like they hurt."

"They do."

"Paul, look at these scratch marks on his forearm."

I notice multiple punctate lesions and redness streaking up and down his arm. "That itch?" I ask.

"Yeah, I think it might be scabies."

"I think so, too. Had it before?"

"Yeah, every time I go to a hospital, it's the same thing."

"We'll need to apply some special lotion—it's called Elimite—to those areas and wash it off in several hours," I explain. "And though I don't see any nits, it might not be a bad idea to give you some permethrin shampoo to kill off any lice that might be sticking around. A precaution."

"Okay," he says, having been through the drill before.

. . .

When I was a medical student at the University of Minnesota in the mid-1980s, a friend and I used to see a man around campus whom we came to call the Bird Man. He could be seen "flying" all over the neighborhood—walking with his shoulders up, his arms slung back, in the manner of a barnyard cock strutting around his pen. Those arms would stay up in that position, and though the man never crowed or clucked, he dressed shabbily, rarely washed himself or his clothes, and rarely said anything except for an occasional howl or yell at nothing in particular. He was not violent. He kept to himself.

In the lexicon of 1950s psychiatry, the Bird Man was an "ambulatory schizophrenic." If you intentionally held your arms up in that takeoff position for more than a few minutes, you would soon be experiencing symptoms of numbness, tingling, and leadenness. But, due to the Bird Man's relative catatonia, a condition of which one element is "waxy flexibility" of the extremities' muscles, his arms could stay in that bizarre position for hours at a time.

If the Bird Man had been wandering around in takeoff position in the 1950s or early 1960s, then he likely would have been residing in some back ward of a state hospital. No doubt he would have been forced to take Thorazine or even to submit to electric shock or insulin coma therapy or a lobotomy. On the back ward, he would have slept in a clean, warm bed, taken hot showers, and been served three reasonably good hot meals a day. He could have watched television or played Ping-Pong or read or gone for walks on the extensive hospital grounds. He could have smoked cigarettes nearly endlessly—in those days ladies' auxiliaries provided cigarette money to indigent psychiatric inmates.

(There are two interesting theories behind the observation that psychiatric patients have historically smoked so much: One is that the nicotine seems to sharpen cognition, at least temporarily. The other is that nicotine induces certain liver enzymes to metabolize psych meds at a faster rate, thereby lessening their effects. The two reasons may be related, since the old psychiatric medications are notorious for causing cognitive dulling.)

In return, the Bird Man would have had to be a "good boy" and not slug any doctors, nurses, orderlies, or peers. He would have had to eschew sex, or at least be very discreet about it, take his meds, and attend group and individual therapy sessions.

The Scottish psychiatrist R. D. Laing, in his 1985 autobiography, *Wisdom, Madness, and Folly,* describes the Bird Men and Ray Shellams of the world and how psychiatrists have been asked to intervene. Laing points out that many members of the public might say something like: "I want that guy out of sight, out of sound, out of mind." He describes these patients when he writes,

> They are not breaking the law, but they arouse in those around them such urgent feelings of pity, worry, fear, disgust, anger, exasperation, concern, that something has to be done. . . . The first, decisive, crunch decision is: should *this* person, or *that* person, be taken away, locked up, and observed for a while?
>
> There is a strange contradiction in society's attitude to psychiatric power. Psychiatrists are empowered by the law of the land. They do not ask for all that has been foisted on them. . . . The hopes placed on [psychiatric power] are unrealistic, the inevitable disillusion unpleasantly nasty. . . .

The autonomy given, indeed imposed on, psychiatry to strip away civil rights and liberties in the name of medical necessity for observation and treatment has no equivalent in any legally authorized power anywhere in our society, except, I suppose, where the torture of prisoners is legal.[2]

Laing began his medical and psychiatric training in the late 1940s and did the bulk of his professional work from the 1950s through the 1970s. It's remarkable how little has changed when you consider what the San Francisco emergency psychiatrist Dr. Bob Buckley has to say about the matter today: "As time goes on, I become more and more aware of how awesome that power is. We're able to just grab people and say, 'You have to be here for seventy-two hours,' with no evidence other than our belief that it's the right thing to do; and we're empowered to do it. We don't have to prove it to anyone. That's a tremendously abusable power. . . . I think I feel comfortable with it because I subject myself to a pretty rigorous interpretation. . . . I feel that, if I don't find myself being buffeted back and forth between the two positions [of releasing or holding a patient], then I'm being too smug in my decision making. I just figure [this buffeting] is a cost of doing business."

By the mid-1980s, after the patients' rights movement and deinstitutionalization—the emptying out of state hospital beds—the Bird Man and other ex-patients like him were now entitled to live out of doors, sleeping in shelter beds in winter and alleyways in summer; to not take any medications or see any social workers or therapists or, God forbid, psychiatrists; and to dine at free-eats places and out of dumpsters. By God, the Bird Man had his freedom, and, there's something to be said for that. But was he "rotting with his rights on"?

The patients' rights movement, which began in the late 1960s and reached a peak in the 1970s and 1980s, came on the scene in response to decades of overly fuzzy commitment laws and an unchecked sense of paternalism among many of the era's psychiatrists. This was an era in which diagnoses and treatment goals were vague, psychoanalysts were kings, and long-term commitments were the norm. Psychiatrists wielded too much power.

"The way the old laws were drafted was pretty broad. In order to be committed by a judge, the patient only had to be deemed mentally ill and in need of care, treatment, restraint. It was kind of vague. The criteria were pretty general. A lot of people could fit into that category pretty easily," says Dr. Isadore Talesnick, a man of extraordinary decency, pragmatism, and moderation and a colleague of mine who began his career in the 1950s and still practices psychiatry in the twenty-first century. "A family member could petition for it under the old law. But once a person was committed, there wasn't a time limit. It was up to the clinical people to decide when someone was ready to be discharged. And that was too long. It was abused in some places. So it had to be changed. It *had* to be changed."

The federal Community Mental Health Centers Act was passed under the supervision of President John F. Kennedy in 1963. According to T. M. Luhrmann, "The initiative had established community mental health centers, which were to treat psychiatric problems locally and preemptively, so that the hospitalized could return to their families and those at risk would not get so sick. . . . The money never really materialized, but many of the hospitalized were released from hospitals despite the lack of community care."[3]

In California in 1958, about 37,500 patients were hospitalized in ten state mental hospitals. Thirty years later, approximately 6,000 patients resided in four state hospitals. An estimated 20,000 to 30,000 patients were homeless in the state of California in the late 1980s.[4] "Because the infrastructure of community mental health care was never established, homelessness became the only option for many of the former patients," writes Luhrmann.[5]

"During Ronald Reagan's administration as governor of California, six of the state hospitals were closed," says Dr. Talesnick. "So it was a pretty quick emptying out. I've often thought, 'Who knows what happened to some of those patients?'" It is probably fair to say that many of them became homeless, died, or were incarcerated. Not only did psychiatrists begin seeing more patients out in the community, but they were also seeing sicker and sicker patients, many of whom just a few years earlier would have been taken care of in state hospitals. It's not too big a stretch to posit that the explosion of hardcore drug abuse and infectious disease transmission of the 1980s and after was at least partially due to this dehospitalization.[6]

New mental health laws, which provided due-process standards in the rules governing involuntary commitment, were passed in California in 1967. These laws, referred to as LPS laws, corresponding to the three state representatives—Lanterman, Petris, and Short—who sponsored the legislation, were fully operational by 1972. These state laws established the grounds for a seventy-two-hour involuntary commitment based on the criteria of danger to self, danger to others, and grave disability.

Dr. Talesnick recalls the atmosphere of the 1970s and also the early years of the hearings, which in those days were presided over by full-fledged judges. "In California, and in [the San Francisco Bay Area] particularly, there was a lot of patient agitation about involuntary hospitalization and medication. There was always a paranoid tinge to it, but at the same time there was always a kernel of truth somewhere in it. That was a difficult time. You were defending things that you weren't really happy with yourself. You weren't happy with everything about the medications; you weren't happy with everything about involuntary hospitalization. But you did what you thought you could do. I used to go to court a lot the first two or three years of LPS. I felt strongly that some people needed treatment, needed to stay in the hospital. I was kind of gung ho to fight this. It was an interesting time, a little crazy too." The tenor and the occasionally acrimonious nature of the hearings as described by Dr. Talesnick are similar to what I experienced in 1989 when I was a psychiatric resident working on the locked ward at San Francisco General Hospital.

Today, an involuntary patient has no legal recourse when detained under section 5150. If a doctor and hospital choose to petition for an additional fourteen-day involuntary commitment, a 5250 in LPS parlance, then at that time the patient has the right to request a legal hearing to present his or her case against being further confined in the hospital. The legal question is framed in these terms: Does "probable cause" exist that would allow the doctor and hospital to continue holding the person involuntarily?

A hearing officer comes to the hospital and listens to the doctor's side and then the patient's side of the story. The doctor, representing the hospital, explains the rationale for continuing to hold the patient. The patient tries to convince the hearing officer that he or she should be released. Though it is a civil court hearing, the patient has the right to be represented by an attorney. Most use the services of a public defender from the mental health court. The hospital and doctor do not have counsel at the hearing.

As the doctor representing the hospital, I often felt like a jailer, sometimes justifiably so, sometimes not. I would prepare at length for the hearings I felt strongly about, and in fact I came to relish the challenge of trying to outduel the public defender and to sway the court's hearing officer.

In the watershed 1976 case *O'Connor v. Donaldson,* the United States Supreme Court "ruled that harmless mentally ill patients cannot be confined against their will without treatment if they can survive outside. According to the Court, a finding of mental illness alone cannot justify a state's confining persons in a hospital against their will. Instead, involuntarily confined patients must be considered dangerous to themselves or others or possibly so unable to care for themselves that they cannot survive outside."[7]

Psychiatrists were now charged with a duty to maintain public safety, a responsibility more consistent with police powers than with medical ones. The task of a psychiatrist, which previously involved evaluating a person's need for treatment, had shifted suddenly to that of establishing "dangerousness criteria" and attempting to predict who might constitute a danger to self or a danger to others. Where once the state had endeavored to take responsibility for patients unable to care for themselves, it now took the role of preventing harm to society. Subsequent legal cases built stronger and stronger safeguards around a patient's right to refuse treatment, so that more and more the burden of proof—that a patient needed to be confined and treated—fell to the increasingly beleaguered psychiatrists.

At the same time, evolving judicial precedents more or less announced that psychiatrists should be able to foresee "preventable" acts of suicide or violence. It became our job to somehow keep those dangerous people locked up, preventing self-harm and mayhem. I refer to this as the crystal ball standard.

It is a plainly unfortunate fact that changes in psychiatric practice over the years have been driven much more by political, legal, fiscal, and regulatory factors than by any particular advances in scientific evidence, ideally derived from the gold standard of randomized, double-blind, placebo-controlled research. The state of the art has been summarized by an expert consensus guide called *Treatment of Behavioral Emergencies,* which was generated by surveying fifty experts in emergency psychiatry:

> Behavioral emergencies are a common and serious problem for consumers, their communities, and the healthcare settings on which they rely to contain, assess, and ultimately help the individual in a behavioral crisis. Partly because of the inherent dangers of this situation, there is little research to guide provider responses to this challenge. Key constructs such as agitation have not been adequately operationalized so that the criteria defining a behavioral emergency are vague. The significant progress that has been made for some disease states with better treatments and higher consumer acceptance has not penetrated this area of practice.[8]

The practice of emergency and acute care psychiatry is more highly influenced today by health-care policy makers, insurance and pharmaceutical companies, regulators, activists, and lawyers than it is by those who actually provide the care—namely, psychiatrists, psychologists, psychiatric nurses, nurse practitioners, social workers, pharmacists, and occupational therapists. Acute care psychiatrists today work in a system limited by the following realities:

It's become much harder to keep patients, who are often in desperate need of treatment, in the hospital long enough to adequately stabilize them. Either they prevail at their hearings and win release from the hospital, or the insurance providers (including MediCal and MediCare) decertify care, meaning they stop paying for the provision of care, putting the hospital in the delicate position of not getting paid for it.

It's still nearly impossible to predict suicides, assaults, or homicides—legal opinions notwithstanding. Lawsuits, though relatively rare, are still filed against psychiatrists for wrongful deaths.

It's become very difficult to place the extremely mentally ill, who actually do need long-term psychiatric care, behind the locked doors of a state hospital.

It requires much more effort these days to make people take their medications, the irony being that this era's pharmacopoeia is much less toxic and much more humane compared to the old standard-bearers Thorazine and Haldol.

The pendulum has swung a bit in the twenty-first century to the point that we are now at least asking the question "Should an individual patient have as much right to treatment as he or she has the right to refuse treatment?" But, alas, treatment costs money. It's become convenient for cynical advocates of "no new taxes," and for politicians and government bean-counters, to ally themselves with impassioned advocates of individual freedom who champion a person's right to refuse treatment rather than a person's right to treatment.

Although the state of California passed legislation in 2001 that made involuntary outpatient mental health treatment legal in certain situations, it also made the new law bureaucratically onerous for California counties to administer, and, to add insult to injury, it failed to authorize additional funds for implementation. Not surprisingly, the law, unworkable as it is, has never been applied in San Francisco, at least as of 2009. Lengths of stay for hospitalized patients continue to shrink. The revolving door between admissions and discharges spins faster and faster.

. . .

"When did you last have a regular place to stay?" I ask Mr. Shellam.

"'Bout ten years ago. The Civic Center Hotel. Then I lost my SSI and got kicked out, because I couldn't afford it no more. Been out on the streets ever since." ("SSI" stands for Supplemental Security Income.)

"What's it like out there for you?"

"Well, it's gotten a little worse the last couple of years, but I prefer it to the shelters."

"Why?"

"Mostly I don't like bein' around all those people. All that coughin' and crack smokin'. It's kinda dangerous. Might get TB, might get beat up. I'd rather take my chances in the alley; at least I got a cop walkin' by me a few times a night."

"Anything else?"

"Yeah, doc, they kick you out at six A.M.; can't come back 'til four in the afternoon. I just got to drag my shit around for ten hours and then bring it back to the shelter, where it might get ripped off anyway."

"You know, Ray, what you say makes a lot of sense. But what I don't get is why you let your hygiene get so bad, why you don't take a shower more often."

Mr. Shellam pauses. He looks up at me expectantly. "I dunno. I guess it just don't bother me."

"Is it because there's nowhere to wash your clothes, take a shower?"

"Naw, I can usually find a shower in a shelter or, worst comes to worst, take one over at Martin's," he says, referring to a San Francisco charity mainstay, Martin de Porres, on the South of Market end of Potrero Avenue.

"And your clothes?"

"Well, doc," Mr. Shellam starts sheepishly, "that's easy. I usually panhandle just enough to get drunk. I s'pose I could use my change to do my laundry, but once I get drunk about 10 or 11 in the morning, my only focus is to stay drunk 'til I pass out later in the day."

"How 'bout food?"

"Sometimes I eat lunch at St. Anthony's, you know, one meal a day, but . . ." His voice trails off.

"But what?" I ask.

"But I'm usually drunk by then, so I skip it. Sometimes I'll dig some food out of a garbage can. You'd be surprised at how much those yuppies leave in the can," he says, referring to the legions of suits and skirts who work in San Francisco's Financial District, which abuts our version of skid row, the Tenderloin and South of Market.

"And what do you drink?"

"Steel Reserve."

"Rotgut Steelies, eh?" I chide.

The mention of his beverage of choice brings a smile to his lips. "Yeah, doc, Steelies. Just a buck out the door."

We're talking Steel Reserve High Gravity Lager in a can: a.k.a. 211, the medieval sign for steel, also the California penal code section for robbery. It's twenty-four ounces of malt liquor, which has the viscosity of 5W-30 motor oil and a faintly sweet scent, like that of watered-down maple syrup. At many convenience stores and neighborhood markets, a can costs ninety-two cents before taxes—"just a buck out the door"—and, at 8.1 percent alcohol, packs nearly the wallop of four regular twelve-ounce beers. Now slam down three or four of those, and you'll be keeping your old pal delirium tremens at bay for another day or two. Seeing as how one can rustle up four bucks spare-changing in an hour or two, is it any wonder that these dyed-in-the-wool alcoholics—who often fall down, seize, soil themselves, get hypothermia, get assaulted, get rolled, get belligerent with tourists, and occasionally walk naked into traffic—never get sober?

"Ray, how many cans do you drink in an average day?"

"As many as I can afford 'til I pass out."

"How many does it take?"

"Oh, I don't know. Six? Seven?" To get an idea of what this means, consider that this amount of alcohol is equivalent to about a case of regular beer a day.

"When'd you last have a taste?"

"Yesterday, maybe four in the afternoon."

His hands, betraying him, shake ever so slightly, and a few beads of sweat have formed on his nose. His blood pressure is up, systolic 170 over diastolic 105, and his heart is racing at 114 beats per minute.

"Do you have a history of high blood pressure? Are you supposed to be on pills for it?"

"No, not that I know."

"You detox hard? Do you get alcohol-withdrawal seizures? Convulsions?"

"Naw, just the shakes, real bad."

"Ever see snakes or get superparanoid when you detox?"

"Just once, but I was okay."

Ray Shellam, with his sweating, tremors, high blood pressure, and rapid heart rate, is a textbook example of a man on the brink of at least a moderate bout of what I've come to call garden-variety alcohol withdrawal, complicated by a moderate amount of dehydration.

The treatment for alcohol withdrawal, which we see routinely in psych emergency, is water, food, vitamins, and specific medications to forestall seizures and the more dreaded but rarely seen delirium tremens. Physicians generally prescribe benzodiazepines, also known as "benzos," which are sedatives, or minor tranquilizers such as Valium and its cousins Librium, Ativan, and Klonopin, to safely detox a patient who's gone off of alcohol.

"We're going to monitor and treat you for alcohol withdrawal, Ray. We'll give you some vitamins and some Ativan. Have you ever been in residential alcohol treatment?"

Mr. Shellam looks down and sheepishly mutters, "No."

Though highly skeptical and almost certain of what his answer will be, I ask, "Do you have any interest in going to residential alcohol treatment?"

"Well, doc," he says, and then pauses, seemingly not wanting to hurt my feelings, "let me think about that."

In the parlance of the street-dwelling alcoholics of the world, that's a screaming "NO!" Mr. Shellam doesn't seem to mind getting cleaned up, getting some real food, getting detoxed, and spending the night, but I sense he'll want out of psych emergency in the morning. I continue my evaluation.

"Other than when you've been here, have you ever seen a psychiatrist?"

"Yeah, but that was years ago. I was going to college, and in my junior year I had a nervous breakdown. It was awful. They committed me to the hospital and shot me up with Haldol. I was on monthly shots for a few years, but then my mouth started moving around and the doctors got scared and took me off of it. I felt so much better. That stuff had me feeling like a zombie, all stiff and slowed down. That was when I decided to come to San Francisco, to get a little change of scenery. I've mostly flown under the radar since I moved here from Omaha. Something I really like about it here. People don't hassle you for being different."

Some patients with chronic schizophrenia demonstrate heedlessness in performing basic personal hygiene and can suffer global self-neglect. This does not seem to reflect a conscious decision to employ slack habits of self-care, but rather seems to be a feature of the illness that can almost come to define them. Now, if you or I didn't shower for three days, we'd say, "Hey, I feel grimy; I need to clean up." But many of these patients don't even seem to notice their condition.

"But don't you want help?" I sputter. "Don't you want to get off the streets, have a place to get clean, wash your clothes, to eat?"

"Naw, I like my freedom. I don't like being cooped up. The hotel was okay, but I like the street better. There's always somethin' goin' on."

"But don't you feel like the street's a dangerous place?"

"Safer than those damn fleabag SROs they got around here. Filled up with hookers, drug addicts, all sorts of bad people. Locked up in your room with some psycho pounding on your door, threatening you for five dollars. Out here, the police is here, there's always help to be had. I'd rather take my chances in the out-of-doors."

I find myself really liking Ray Shellam. He is one of those salt-of-the-earth characters that I know well from my years growing up and living in Minnesota. Not an ounce of guile. No manipulating. No threats. I make routine inquiries about active psychotic symptoms, such as paranoid or grandiose delusions or hallucinations, and he is manifesting none of these.

In an ideal world I would have a chance to review his original medical records from his college days, twenty-plus years earlier, to see for myself whether a diagnosis of schizophrenia actually applies to him. But it's plain to me that, at this point, he has no acute symptoms of psychosis except for, perhaps, what led the officers to bring him to psych emergency in the first place: his almost wanton disregard for his hygiene, his avariciousness for alcohol at the expense of his basic needs, and his, well, unsightliness in the eyes of San Francisco's Chamber of Commerce.

It's likely that in college he had a bona fide "nervous breakdown," sanitized shorthand for a first episode of psychosis that may or may not have become chronic. For the sake of argument, let's say that he did have schizophrenia. Then the type of schizophrenia he suffers from now would be more precisely called either a "residual" or an "undifferentiated" type. In laypersons' terms, his acute psychotic symptoms went into remission.

What he's left with these days are a few of the so-called negative symptoms—disorganized thinking or behavior, poor judgment, social isolation, and the aforementioned neglect of basic self-care.

Dr. Buckley has this to say about the Ray Shellams of the world who are brought to his doorstep for evaluation: "You can probably let this guy go, and he's not going to die right away. To a lot of those guys I say, 'You might not need to be here, but I sure wish you'd go to a clinic, see a social worker, or something.' They're telling me that they're functioning, but they don't look like they're functioning. There are times when I just say, 'I wouldn't want my daughter or my son or my brother or my cousin to be living like this, and I don't think this guy's mother or father or brothers or sisters would want him living like this. And maybe I'm wrong, and maybe I shouldn't do this, but I can't bring myself to let this person go.'

"It probably shouldn't, but it does, involve how desperately they don't want to be in the hospital," remarks Dr. Buckley. "It probably shouldn't be, but it is, affected by my second-guessing of the legal system, by my thinking that the court will probably let this guy go in a few days anyway. Or by my thinking: 'I'm not letting this guy go; I'll let the judge decide.' It's not part of a really elegant solution to the problem."

. . .

Before checking in with Mr. Shellam the next morning, I take a look at the medication order book and note that he has received a delousing, vitamins, and no less than ten milligrams of lorazepam overnight to prevent him from seizing or going into DTs from his alcohol withdrawal.

I find him dressed in a hospital gown, picking through items on the hospital's cart of volunteered clothing. This is a necessity because his own clothes were sent away in a red bag marked for incineration to kill all the cooties and germs they no doubt had accumulated. Mr. Shellam still sports a tangled beard, but his hair is freshly washed and parted down the middle. He greets me with a smile. "Mornin', doc. Just pickin' out a new set of duds here. Guess my other ones was radioactive."

The tremor is gone. The sweating has dissipated. It's been more than thirty-six hours since his last drink, and he's looking pretty good.

"Hold out your hands for me," I say. "Yeah, straight out like that. Did you eat breakfast this morning?"

"Yeah, scrambled eggs."

"Any nausea, vomiting, seeing things?"

"Just you, doc."

"Any thoughts about wantin' to kill yourself or hurt anyone else?"

"Naw, you know that." Which indeed I do.

"Hey, now that I've eaten and gotten some new clothes, when can I get out of here?"

It's amazing how good these guys can look after an old-fashioned hose-down, some new clothes, and a day or so off the sauce. Maybe a little bewildered, but unfailingly polite and cooperative, and usually with no evidence of a chronic psychotic or mood disorder. And invariably, after a good cleanup and "three-hots-and-a-cot," they are thirsty—*very, very* thirsty. We're not talking Coca-Cola here. They can get a little cranky if you decide to keep them in lockdown too long.

"Well, I don't know, Ray, you were in an awfully sorry state when you got here yesterday. You looked and smelled like crap," I say. I feel frustrated, so I lay it on pretty thick. "How am I supposed to believe that you won't get that way again in just a few weeks? That's no way to live." I can see Mr. Shellam drinking himself to death in the next few years, and I don't like the looks of it.

"Well, I'd be willing to go to a shelter, go to AA, try to stop drinkin'."

As much as I want to believe him, I don't think he'll make it. "What about residential treatment, Ray? I don't know if I can get you in, but we can at least try."

"No, I'd rather do it as an outpatient."

My heart sinks. I know that these responses—which I no more believe than I presume the earth is flat—would easily persuade a hearing officer of the mental health court to let Mr. Shellam leave the hospital if I were to invoke code 5250, citing his "grave disability," and admit him to a locked psychiatric ward. Even if his (nonexistent) family or his (nonexistent) primary care doctor or his friends (drinking buddies) want him locked up in a hospital to prevent him from drinking and to get him back on track, the necessary political will and financial resources are simply not there. If I were to admit him, he would certainly be discharged in a few days, one way or the other, and despite a quick cleanup, he would once again most likely return to a life of dumpster diving, Steel Reserve swilling, and Levi's layering. As one veteran nurse in psych emergency commented when discussing a similar case, "This place is like an expensive car wash. Like that one over there: he paid his five bucks, he's been scrubbed, so now you just send his ass back out there."

"Good-bye, Mr. Shellam. Now I don't want to see you back here anytime soon. And I sure as hell don't want to see you spare-changin' down on Market Street."

"Don't worry, doc, tomorrow's check day. I should be good to go for at least a few days."

"Good luck, sir, and may God bless you."

I wave good-bye.

THE JURY

Playing the Suicide Card

Rick Demerit stands in front of me, swaying, glassy-eyed, smelling of cheap vodka, the hardcore alcoholic's favorite drink next to Steel Reserve. He occasionally mumbles and laughs to himself as he stands at a sort of attention in front of the triage desk, which is located just inside the front door of psych emergency.

The ambient lights are turned down low, seeing as how it's only 7:45 A.M. and many of the patients are just waking up, asking for breakfast. He's been brought in by the SFPD for threatening to kill himself after the police were called to check out what sounded like a domestic disturbance in a room at a flophouse hotel, one of dozens in the TL. Rick's arms are behind him, his wrists in handcuffs.

It's not too bad a day in psych emergency. Only about fifteen cases are listed on the board, only two of the four seclusion rooms are in use, only one manic patient is careening around the clinic, refusing medications and stopping just short of the threshold at which we could medicate her against her will. As the triage nurse and I talk to the police and Mr. Demerit, the manic woman whizzes by us a few times, praying and grimacing. "Yessiree,

Bob, I am overdue for a day out shopping," she whispers to one of her voices.

"Any problems bringing him in, officer?" asks Maureen, the triage nurse.

"No, he's been a real gentleman," says one officer, a tall, muscular, mustachioed white man with a clean-shaven head. He wears the timeless "Officer Murphy" cap of a beat cop.

"But he sure likes to talk a lot, " says the other officer, a petite Filipina. "It was kinda drivin' us nuts, to be honest. Glad we're here."

"Ma'am, these police officers have been very nice to me," says Rick Demerit, his mouth agape, his words slurry. He has brown tousled hair and sports the five o'clock shadow of a young turk. He wears blue denims, a white T-shirt, and a brown leather bomber jacket. His maroon Converse Chuck Taylor high-top shoes are worn but clean.

"Have you been drinking?" I ask.

"Oh, yes, sir, I'm an alcoholic. I drink two pints of vodka almost every day. Sometimes more. If I don't drink, I get the shakes real bad."

Rick is searched by one of our psychiatric technicians. The contents of his pockets spill onto the desk. It's the usual—keys, change, a few crumpled bills, scraps of notes-to-self. From one of his coat pockets, however, comes an empty pint bottle of Royal Gate Vodka, and, voilà, two small white powdery clumps wrapped in aluminum foil and a small glass pipe.

The female cop snatches the pipe and the presumed crack cocaine. "I'll get rid of these for you," she says.

"That'd be nice," says sassy Maureen, not missing a beat, straight outta Brooklyn. "No wonder the dude's so happy. A few uppers with your downers makes for an all-arounder, huh?"

"I guess we didn't search him so well," says the officer, mildly apologetic. What? You can interface with a cop in San Francisco with a couple rocks of crack cocaine and paraphernalia in your pocket and not go to jail? Not even a misdemeanor ticket for possession? Apparently not. Welcome to San Francisco! It's not Mayberry. Crack cocaine is so prevalent in the TL, in fact, that I think someone would have to be packing a large bundle of it to get booked into jail on a charge of felony possession with intent to sell.

Rick stands by politely, not talking, a sloppy grin on his face as he looks around psych emergency. "Would you remove these handcuffs, please?" he asks.

"Are you going to be in control of your behavior here?" asks Maureen. "Can we trust you?"

"Oh, yes, ma'am, by all means," he says.

"Well, okay, Rick. You do seem like a happy drunk."

An officer unlocks his handcuffs and Rick stumbles toward one of two enormous, blocky blue chairs—measuring about four feet by four feet by four feet and made of hard plastic—the closest thing to a waiting room that psych emergency has to offer. The Fred Flintstone chairs are too heavy to throw across the room. Though many have tried, only a very few have even gotten these bad boys off the floor.

The manic woman briefly perches next to Mr. Demerit, who studiously (and wisely) ignores her. She flits skyward and is on her way, once again purposelessly wandering about the place.

"So what's the story, officers?" asks Maureen.

"Oh, yeah, well, the call came from the TL—the usual, a disturbance in a hotel room. The manager called 911 because there was screaming and shouting and the sound of furniture break-ing in there. The manager seemed like he was used to it—it was one of the worst hotels down at Turk and Geary—but I guess he had been getting complaints from some of the other paying cus-tomers. And when we got in the room, Mr. Demerit was crying, saying he'd been off his meds and that he was going to kill him-self. We determined then that he was a danger to himself."

"Any evidence of DV?" I ask, using the shorthand for domes-tic violence.

"No, the woman did not have any marks or bruises, and she denied any physical violence at the hands of Mr. Demerit."

"Did you check his rap sheet, officer?" I ask. "Any war-rants?"

"We did, and he has some priors but no outstanding warrants," says the male officer. "He's got a trial date next week. I was actu-ally hoping to find a warrant so we could take him to jail."

"You mean, a couple rocks, a pipe in his possession? That's not enough to book him?"

"Well, yeah, but he'd get out OR'd in a day or two, since it's a misdemeanor and the jail's so crowded. Plus, you know how the jail nurses feel about receiving a suicidal patient."

"Yes, officer, I do know," I say. "Fair enough.

"Thanks, doc," he says.

"Okay, officers, thank you," says Maureen. "Just make sure you fill in all the blanks on the 5150 form, and then you're on your way."

I don't want to challenge the cop too much for not arresting Rick Demerit on the spot. But I think they brought him to us this morning because it means a hell of a lot less paperwork for them.

The two police officers give us a wave, a smile, and a wink and thank us before leaving. They've got a job that I wouldn't want, but I know for a fact, because many of them have told me, that they feel the same way about our jobs.

. . .

People seek help for a wide variety of personal reasons. Most patients come to psych emergency with no ulterior motive. Most folks just want help dealing with their depression, their psychosis, or their addictions and aren't really looking to pull any fast ones. But claiming or exaggerating suicidal thoughts and plans has come to be seen as one of the few reliable tickets for admission to the hospital, or at least for an overnight cleanup in psych emergency. According to Ross D. Ellenhorn, a social worker, psychotherapist, sociologist, and the author of *Parasuicidality and Paradox: Breaking through the Medical Model,* this kind of help-seeking behavior is a direct effect of what's called the medicalization of mental illness.

Classifying psychiatric illnesses as medical problems has accomplished several things, many of them useful. It has established a system of psychiatric diagnosis, formalized treatment approaches, reduced stigma for family members of the psychiatrically ill, and correctly identified the genetic and biomedical components of many major mental illnesses, such as schizophrenia, bipolar disorder, major depression, and severe anxiety disorders. However, it has done little to clarify the diagnosis and treatment of the many personality-disordered patients who are often described as manipulative, gamey, or malingering. And in tandem with the judicial precedents that have given psychiatrists the unenviable task of trying to predict dangerousness, the medicalization of mental illness has produced a notable unintended consequence. It has helped to create a small but significant class of professional patients who have learned to play the suicide card to obtain services. "Indeed," says Ellenhorn, "patienthood would not exist without clinicians who readily view the world through the medical model. . . . Parasuicidality [is] . . . a symptom of the pervasive use of a medical worldview to define and respond to human behavior."[1]

The term *parasuicidality* was created to describe the behavior of a subset of individuals who continually threaten to commit suicide or who cut themselves or take small overdoses in order to assume the role of patient, not with the intention of dying by such acts. Ellenhorn has identified suicidal threats and gestures as occurring within a sociological perspective in which patients are merely taking on a role created by society, its institutions, and its system of tort liability and jurisprudence. Ellenhorn calls "the perpetual access of this role a patient career or patienthood. . . . This role protects individuals from certain painful psychological experiences." He goes on to say, "Parasuicidality . . . typically leads to an institutional response, for it is most often followed by a clinical intervention. . . . I see parasuicidal behavior as a means some individuals use to access a kind of interaction and a type of social role that can only be achieved through a relationship with clinical professionals."[2]

These days, as the economy tanks, substance abuse in the community takes off, and housing gets ever more expensive, a sizable number of patients are coming to psych emergency with a specific agenda. The three most common items on the helpseeker's wish list? To be taken care of, ideally forever; to avoid bad stuff, like jail time; and to get good stuff, like sedating drugs and free housing. Patients such as these eat up a lot of time, money, energy, and patience in a system busting at the seams, because they do not get discouraged easily, coming back again and again and again. Their inappropriate pursuit of services can deprive patients who are not out on a hustle.

The crustiest old-timers on staff in psych emergency do not want to give these folks anything; they do not want to make things too comfortable for them; they do not want them coming back. But even the more compassionate, less-burned-out nurses who work the triage desk have their breaking points. As one said recently at 7:30 A.M., before his shift started in earnest, "I'm not gonna let myself get scammed today. There are too many scammers out there."

Cynicism is a morale killer, but a bit of skepticism is a healthy thing. My attempt at a solution to the problem has always been: if you can give something to patients that legitimately meets their needs, something not overly gratifying or unreasonable, then you should do that, and perhaps they won't have to keep coming back. This stance generally helps me to avoid burnout.

My colleague Dr. Bob Buckley asks a rhetorical question: "Who wants *care,* literally to be taken care of, but who might be better off in the long run making their *own* way out in the community?" He explained that in the early 1980s, when he worked in a residential program in community mental health, most of his patients were people with chronic psychotic disorders who had recently left state hospitals. He noticed that within a year or two, however, most of the new patients entering the program were less psychiatrically ill. "The patient load was becoming more and more personality-disordered people and drug addicts, who were much more vocal and demanding than the chronic schizophrenics, who were out shuffling along the sidewalks. How big should the safety net be? How easy should it be to get stuff? What should we do about this?"

The distinction between the two patient groups is important. It is easy to see someone with schizophrenia as suffering from an illness that is no fault of his or her own. Conversely, it's been assumed over the years that people with personality disorders, alcoholism, and addiction have more control over their conditions. In reality, these patients are likely also suffering from a disorder of the brain, a problem in hardwiring, if you will, that might make it difficult for them to control their maladaptive behaviors. It's just that medical scientists do not understand these illnesses as well as they do schizophrenia. But it is undeniable that a handful of patients feel entitled to have it *their* way or no way at all.

This phenomenon can be understood from two different historical sources—one an unintended consequence of the changes in involuntary commitment laws over the years, and the other a reflection of the long-standing conflict between "good government" idealists and "libertarian" cynics. As mentioned in the previous chapter, in the 1960s and 1970s, decisions in the courtroom directed psychiatrists to focus less on providing care to the sickest patients based on their actual need for treatment, and to focus more on somehow predicting dangerousness, with the goal of preventing suicide or violence.

The writings of Charlotte Towle, a liberal American social worker of the mid-twentieth century, and Theodore Dalrymple, a conservative British psychiatrist of the modern era, typify the acrimonious history of this issue of entitlements. In the United States, shortly after World War II, the forerunner of the Social Security system, called the Family Security Agency, was created. In 1945, Towle wrote the first edition of a book called *Common Human Needs*, a guide for the nation's eligibility workers that was designed to help them better understand the disabled and sick people who would be applying for benefits throughout the country.

For a variety of reasons, her book set off a political firestorm. The book became a bogeyman for McCarthyites. Conservative legislators and pundits associated Towle's use of the word *socialized* (as in children being "socialized" to be respectful, responsible individuals) with the concept of socialism. These folks fired allegations at her, asserting that her creation of a "socialized state" inappropriately promoted a socialist system of government. According to Towle:

> This matter of the individual's right to assistance currently is feared by some people, to whom it connotes indiscriminate giving to any and every idler who chooses to be supported by those who toil. It is even decried as a threat to democracy. . . . [It is feared] that when man is accorded the opportunity to survive, he not only will come to feel entitled to depend on others for support but also to expect a way of life beyond a bare survival level.
>
> We live in a period of scientific enlightenment and of great technical achievement which, if intelligently used, could render the life of all people more satisfactory than ever before.[3]

Leading the modern-day charge against this progressive idealism is the pseudonymous Dalrymple, whose series of columns in the London newspaper the *Spectator* formed the basis of his book *Life at the Bottom: The Worldview That Makes the Underclass.* Dalrymple says:

> We are constantly told by those liberals whose nostrums of the past have contributed so richly to this wretched situation that

society (by which is meant government) should do yet more for such pitiable people. But is not homelessness, at least in modern-day society, a special instance of a law first enunciated by a British medical colleague of mine, namely, that misery increases to meet the means available for its alleviation? And does not anti-social behavior increase in proportion to the excuses that intellectuals make for it? . . .

Apologists for nonjudgmentalism point, above all, to its supposed quality of compassion. . . . [A man] never asks where his fellow man's suffering comes from, whether it be self-inflicted or not: for whatever reason, he sympathizes with it and succors the sufferer.[4]

At least a few times a day in psych emergency, we see a patient whose thought process goes something like this: "How about if I call 911 and tell the operator that I'm gonna kill myself? It's a free ride to the hospital." If the police bring you in on a 5150 hold, you have to undergo a psychiatric assessment before you get released. But if you just walk in to try your luck, you have to talk to the triage nurse, who guards the front door by performing a screening assessment. If a triage nurse allowed every single person who claimed suicidal thoughts and plans into psych emergency, then the place would become overcrowded, figuratively blowing the roof off. Conversely, if a triage nurse turns into "Nurse No" and lets virtually no one in, then bad things, like suicide and violence and instances of individuals getting sicker via neglect, are much more likely to happen. It's a thankless, no-win job.

Imagine yourself for a moment as a homeless person wandering about town in the middle of the night. If it's raining cats and dogs and you don't have money or a charge card to get a hotel room, or you have played the shelter bed lottery and lost, and if you don't want to shiver while trying to sleep under a bridge, fending off rats, thieves, and attackers, then you too will probably think about trying your luck at the triage window. So this is a rational act. I don't blame these folks. I used to get irritated at people bellying up to the desk to get off the streets. But with just a few years of experience, I began to realize that, if I were in the same position, I would probably do the same. Desperate times call for desperate measures.

The person presenting himself or herself at the triage window catches a lot more flies with honey than vinegar. Psychiatric clinicians are human beings, too, and we are more likely to sympathize with a person who seems sincere, authentic, and polite. You don't have to be perfect. We get that you're struggling, and we're working in a place like this to help (or we should be). Most of us are tolerant and understanding (it should be our stock-in-trade) of a wide range of behavior, but if you come across as wanting to be taken care of for the rest of your life, or are seen as jamming us for goodies a little too vigorously, then you will gain little traction.

But this is where it gets tricky. Essentially all these folks, especially the manipulative ones, *do* need some level of assistance for medical and psychiatric care, not to mention food, clothing, and shelter. The question is: Do they require it from a facility where the basic rate is more than one hundred dollars per hour, probably closer to two hundred dollars per hour? Most of them don't.

· · ·

"If it's okay with you, Maureen, I'm going to go interview Mr. Demerit with the new intern here, and then she's going to write up the case."

"Sounds good to me, Dr. Linde. One less case for the nurses."

Maureen finishes taking Rick's vital signs—heart rate and blood pressure are a bit up, which is nothing that a touch of Ativan can't cure. We've got time before he starts to withdraw from the alcohol. He's still got a fair amount of happy juice on board, so the Ativan can wait until after the interview. I introduce the intern and myself to Mr. Demerit and instruct him to follow us to the interview room, where we take our respective seats. He does so wordlessly, which I find curious since he was so loquacious with Maureen and the cops.

I start, as I do with most patients, with an open-ended approach. "As I mentioned before, my name is Dr. Linde, and I'm one of the attending psychiatrists here. I wanted to talk to you to see if we could come up with some kind of plan to help you out."

"Yeah, right," he mumbles.

"So, what's been going on in your life lately?"

"You mean, why am I suicidal?" Mr. Demerit sneers.

"That's one way of putting it," I say.

"My life sucks. I'm depressed. I need help." He pauses. "I need to be in the hospital for at least those three days, if not a week or two."

I sense his irritability, lack of candor, and laser vision for getting admitted to the hospital. I continue with the open-ended approach. "What is making you depressed these days, do you think?"

"Are you listening or what? I told you. My life sucks. I'm depressed."

"It might help to talk a little bit about what's actually going on in your life. For example, how are things going in your relationship?"

"Don't patronize me, doc. My life sucks. I'm depressed and I'm suicidal. I need to be in the hospital."

I decide on switching to a more closed-end approach because of Mr. Demerit's repetitions, which only make him seem vague and evasive. "Is it true what the police officer is saying? Have you been thinking about hurting yourself?"

"Oh, yes, sir, I'm a danger to myself and others."

"Have you ever been a patient here?"

"I don't believe so."

"Are you on psych meds?"

"What, you don't think I'm crazy, do you?"

"Never said you were. Never said you were."

"I'm not crazy," he says. "I'm suicidal. I came here for my three days—it's a seventy-two-hour hold, isn't it?"

"Yes, the 5150 hold is for *up* to seventy-two hours, but that doesn't mean you'll be staying here that long. We're only supposed to hold people for twenty-four hours here. If you still need to be here after twenty-four hours, then you might get admitted to the psych ward."

"You think I can get admitted? That would be great." His eyes brighten. "Doctor, I'm very suicidal. I'm sure I'll need to be admitted."

"We'll see," I say. "We'll do a formal evaluation and then observe you over a period of time. If we feel that you're at risk of suicide, then we'll admit you to the hospital. You ever see a psych before?" I use the jail and prison shorthand for "mental health professional."

"I'm not sure what you mean."

"What I mean is, have you ever been seen by a psychiatrist, psychologist, therapist, anything like that?"

His brow furrows, his face reddens, the glow disappears. "You can stop asking me these stupid-ass questions now," he says, going from obsequious to sarcastic to hostile in a matter of seconds. "Don't think you're such a fuckin' whiz kid!"

"Hey, what happened? We need to do an evaluation to figure out how we can try to help you."

"Hey, I need my meds. That would help."

"And what are they?"

"Well, Vicodin, 'cuz I've got a chronic pain syndrome, you see, and Klonopin for my seizures, and Valium, as I've got a little anger management problem. Oh, and medical marijuana."

"Do you have pain right now?"

"Yeah, I always have pain. My whole body hurts. Eleven out of ten."

"Were you in an accident?"

"Can't you read my fuckin' chart? Yes, I've been in a few. I had a motorcycle accident. I broke every fuckin' bone in my body."

"How many Vikes you want?"

"I usually take two Extra Strength every four hours. And I'm on Klonopin, two milligrams three times a day; Valium, twenty milligrams four times a day."

"I can order all that stuff, probably not *both* the Klonopin and Valium, though, since they are essentially the same medication."

"All right, all right." He seems to calm down a bit.

"What about the crack?" I ask.

"I don't smoke every day, but I pretty much smoked all night long. Why you think I only got two rocks left?" He smiles.

"Yeah, pretty smart to smoke all the evidence," I say.

"Hey, thanks, doc," he says. "Then I start drinkin' to come down."

"Jeez, how do you get the money for all that?"

"Well, I'm on SSI."

"Sure, which would take you through only a few days at that rate."

"I don't smoke like that every day, you know, but I do see your point."

"How 'bout the rest of the money?"

"Hah, you have a lot of nerve. Let's just say I'm a small businessman. Entrepreneurship—it's an American ideal."

"Sure," I say. I speculate that he's a midlevel drug dealer or a fence, and not a bad one at that if he's never gotten seriously busted.

"So what was goin' on in the hotel room today?"

"I was tryin' to comfort my girlfriend. She got a little upset and started breakin' shit."

"Did she hit you?"

"Yeah, she was pounding me on my ribs, my guts." He pulls up his shirt and shows me a few fresh bruises on his torso. "Lady got a good punch, don't you think?"

"Did you hit her?"

"I would never hit a lady, doc; what do you take me for?"

"I can't say for sure just yet," I tell him. "So how long have you been feelin' like killing yourself?"

"Oh, it's been goin' on for years—off and on, off and on."

"Have you ever attempted suicide?"

"Well, it depends on how you define suicide."

"Well, have you ever done anything directly to hurt yourself?"

"Does smokin', like, ten rocks in a row until it felt like my head was gonna blow off count?"

"Well, that depends. Were you tryin' to kill yourself with that? Or just get high?"

"What do you think? Of course I was tryin' to kill myself."

"Engaging in any other high-risk activities?"

"Well, let me see, do motorcycle racing, skydiving, fighting as a mercenary count as high-risk enough?"

"Were you hoping you'd die doing any or all of those things?"

His face dims; his voice grows soft; the wise-guy smirk disappears. "Well, not really, but not really caring if I lived either."

"How are you feeling right now?"

His lip curls and his malign stare returns. "You goddamn shrinks with your 'how does that make you feel?' bullshit."

"I noticed you got a little quiet there."

"Don't you go reading too much into things, doc. It didn't mean shit."

I don't feel threatened by Mr. Demerit. He reminds me a bit of Jack Nicholson's Randle P. McMurphy character in *One Flew over the Cuckoo's Nest*. "I have a few more questions for you. Have you ever taken an overdose, jumped off a building or bridge, or cut yourself on purpose with a knife?"

"None of those."

"Have you ever held a loaded gun to your head?"

"Not to mine."

"Do you ever see little green men?" I ask. It's one of my mini lie-detector tests for malingering, since this symptom is essentially never reported by a genuinely psychotic person.

"How'd you know?"

"Clinical intuition," I say.

"Yeah, all the time. I can see 'em out of the corner of my eye. They come into my bedroom."

"Well, I've seen your kind of problems before. If you get admitted to the hospital, and that's a pretty big if, your symptoms should be much better in three or four days, after a few doses of Haldol."

"Haldol?" he asks. "No thanks. I've seen that stuff make zombies out of people."

"Well, I can't make you take it, but it might work for you, getting rid of all those little green men."

"You say three or four days?" he asks, his facial features a bit pinched. "I'll need at least a week, I'm sure."

"Well, I don't know how long they'll keep you on the ward if you do get admitted. It'll be up to the psychiatrist up there and the court, of course."

"The court?" he says, a look of panic on his face.

"Don't worry." I smile. "It's not a criminal court. It's the mental health court. I take it you'd like to stay up there for as long as you can."

"Hey, I'm not comin' in here for three hots and a cot, you know. I'm hearin' voices tellin' me to kill myself. I'm a danger to myself. You can't discharge me."

"At a minimum, you'll be staying the night. I'll be back in the morning and we can talk some more."

"I can't wait," he says.

I tuck Rick in for the night with all of his "good" drugs ordered. If nothing else, the medications will prevent him from going into Vicodin or benzodiazepine withdrawal. While the narcotic withdrawal is no more than incredibly uncomfortable, withdrawal from the minor tranquilizers, the benzos, can be potentially life threatening. Between the alcohol still on board, the crack cocaine withdrawal, and his new batch of narcotics and benzos, all of which cause fatigue and sedation, he is bound to sleep well.

. . .

Rick Demerit does not strike me as having what I would call a major mental illness, such as schizophrenia, bipolar disorder, major depression, or a severe anxiety disorder; nonetheless, he is now my patient. He has never been admitted to the psych ward, he isn't taking psych meds, and he did not convincingly demonstrate any symptoms of psychosis, mania, depression, or anxiety. To put it bluntly, he seems to be a moderately adept criminal with a drug problem and a probable personality disorder. He has wangled his way into the hospital in lieu of being booked into jail for possession of drugs and paraphernalia and now may also have a good excuse to miss a future court date.

According to the latest version of the *Diagnostic and Statistical Manual* (DSM-IV-TR), as cited in Kaplan and Sadock, personality disorders are marked by "an enduring pattern of inner experience and behavior that deviates markedly from the expectations of the individual's culture. The pattern is manifested in two (or more) of [the following]: cognition (i.e., ways of perceiving and interpreting self, other people, and events), affectivity (i.e., the range, intensity, lability, and appropriateness of emotional response), interpersonal functioning, (and) impulse control."[5]

The diagnostic bible goes on to say that personality disorders also characterize the "enduring pattern" as "inflexible and pervasive across a broad range of personal and social situations, [and they lead] to clinically significant distress or impairment in social, occupational, or other important areas of functioning." Moreover, "the pattern is stable and of long duration, and its onset can be traced back at least to adolescence or early adulthood."[6]

When you first start out as a psychiatrist, diagnosing a personality disorder can feel like name-calling. The term *personality disorder* is often used pejoratively, reserved for demanding, manipulative, difficult patients. Diagnosing a personality disorder ought to take some time, definitely more than one visit, but archetypes like Rick Demerit pass quickly through psych emergency on a regular basis.

Those who create the most havoc for all health care professionals are the individuals with "cluster B" disorders: the antisocial, borderline, histrionic, and narcissistic. Individuals with "cluster A" disorders, who are paranoid, schizoid, or schizotypal, are similar to persons with schizophrenia. The "cluster C" types are avoidant, dependent, and obsessive-compulsive, which are self-explanatory concepts.

Personality disorders are tricky because they exist near the extreme ends of a spectrum of personality traits. For example, a little paranoia might be good because it helps you to make sound choices regarding your personal safety. But unnecessary suspiciousness will make you vigilant, defensive, and irritable, and this will make you a bit of an outcast.

If you were to consult the DSM-IV-TR and read the personality disorder section, you might find the experience something like reading horoscopes. For example, I don't think I have a personality disorder (frankly, who does?), but I do have a tendency to exhibit dependency, obsessive-compulsive, histrionic, and paranoid traits. Let me see—one from cluster A, one from cluster B, and two from cluster C. It's probably a fairly typical profile for a health care professional. These attributes refer to a broad array of temperamental styles. I hope this personality blend reflects the fact that I'm able to shift and be flexible and call on different strengths when a situation demands it.

Personality disorders are documented as part of a five-category taxonomy by the architects of the DSM, which the American Psychiatric Association and the American Medical Association would prefer that you use when diagnosing a patient. Numeric five-digit codes are assigned to each diagnosis identified in the DSM. Procedure codes are generated in a manual published by the AMA. Insurance companies require a physician to include both diagnostic and procedure codes when submitting a bill for payment. The motivation for organized psychiatry and organized medicine, represented by the APA and the AMA, respectively, for publishing these manuals transcends the academic and theoretical realms and enters into the financial—way into the financial.

A substantial amount of the American Medical Association's revenue comes from the sale of procedural codebooks. Likewise, a large chunk of the American Psychiatric Association's revenue comes from the sales of the latest version of the DSM. (The next generation's diagnostic guidebook, DSM-V, is now being developed, as all its past editions were, by committees of experts. Its estimated publication date is 2012.)

Axis I codes the major psychiatric disorders. Axis II is for the personality disorders and developmental disorders such as mental retardation. Axis III is for medical conditions. Axis IV is for psychosocial stressors. Axis V is now synonymous with the nearly useless (except for billing and mediocre research) Global Assessment of Functioning (GAF) scale, which runs from 0 to 100. Folks assessed as being under 10 on the scale would be naked, grunting, and smearing feces. And I've never met anyone ranking between 90 and 100: they would be shiny, happy Eagle Scouts or Stepford wives who never lie, lust, cheat, or steal, individuals who rarely exist in the natural world.

All the categories get used as shorthand in day-to-day clinical work. When confronted with a personality-disordered patient, one might say, "He has a whiff of Axis II, wouldn't you say?" Or: "Seems like cluster B to me." Or: "Yeah, I GAF'ed him at 39 so we could bill for the visit." Or: "This poor guy is a train wreck; he has multiaxial disease."

Rick Demerit possesses the superficial charm of a sociopath, a brand of antisocial personality disorder. He's just demanding enough to get his needs met, but not over-the-top. He is just endearing enough that I won't boot his ass out the door toot sweet. He is just facile enough in his likely exaggeration of symptoms for me to keep him. Barely.

According to the DSM-IV-TR, "The essential feature of malingering is the intentional production of false or grossly exaggerated physical or psychological symptoms, motivated by external incentives." Malingering is tightly linked to antisocial personality disorder; the DSM-IV-TR defines it as present in an individual with "a pervasive pattern of disregard for and violation of the rights of others occurring since age 15 years, as indicated by three or more of the following criteria: performs criminal acts, demonstrates deceitfulness, impulsivity, irritability, and aggressiveness, reckless disregard for safety, consistent irresponsibility, and lack of remorse."[7]

"These patients often lie; however, believing a patient's lies is not a professional failure. Psychiatrists are trained to detect, understand, and treat psychopathology, not to function as lie detectors. While a certain level of suspicion is essential in the practice of psychiatry, clinicians, determined never to be taken in by deceitful patients, will approach them with such exaggerated suspiciousness that therapeutic work will be impossible."[8]

Theodore Dalrymple works in a hospital's "overdose ward," and he characterizes many of his afflicted patients in these terms: "I'm treated, therefore I am." He says of men who have recently been charged with domestic violence: "They take an overdose for at least one of three reasons, and sometimes for all three: to avoid a court appearance; to apply emotional blackmail to their victims; and to present their own violence as a medical condition that it is the doctor's duty to cure." Dalrymple says he can identify the signals that tell which men are predisposed to beating their partners, the most telling being "a facial expression of concentrated malignity, outraged egotism, and feral suspiciousness— all these give the game away. . . . A man's propensity to violence is as immediately legible in his face and bearing as any other strongly marked character trait."[9]

Though there is some truth to what Dalrymple writes, psychiatrists are better off reserving judgment until they're absolutely certain that they're being conned. I've been fooled dozens of times by what I think are malign stares. It's not until I sit down and actually talk to a patient that I find out what kind of person he or she really is. To believe or not to believe, that is the question. The drug-addicted, alcoholic, personality-disordered Mr. Rick Demerit represents a real-life, real-time, modern-day example of this dilemma.

．　．　．

When I arrive the next day, I hear a report from the day-shift nurse who performed the morning reevaluation of Mr. Demerit.

"He's still saying he's gonna kill himself—get a gun and shoot himself in the head if we let him go," she says. "But he sure looks awful comfortable out there in the dayroom with his pillows, all propped up, holdin' court with a few other patients, sweet-talkin' the younger women in there. He ate a full breakfast, even asked for a second tray. He seems awfully glad to be here. Paul, I say we kick him out. He's a sociopath, a malingerer. I say we call the institutional police and have him escorted out. I don't think he's going to kill himself."

"You know," I say, "I don't think so, either. But he's clutchin' that suicide card awful tight, so it makes it hard for me to let him go."

"I know, I know," sighs the nurse. "You're the doctor. You've got the liability. It's your decision."

"I'll go see him."

The system of medicolegal liability puts responsibility for the prediction of Mr. Demerit's near-term behavior squarely in my hands. In other words, if Rick Demerit gets discharged and succeeds in killing himself, particularly within a day or two, then it automatically becomes my fault. Plus, he'd be dead. I am in the business, after all, of trying to prevent people from killing themselves, even though my task is hampered by the crudeness of the tools of measurement.

I stand off to the side in the dayroom and take a sidelong glance in Mr. Demerit's direction. Sure enough, he is freshly showered, his hair is combed, and he's grinning from ear to ear as he flirts with a twenty-something Asian woman who is here because she took an overdose. I approach him. Despite his seeing me, his demeanor does not appreciably change. "Good morning, Mr. Demerit."

"Hi, doc."

"Could we go talk in private for a little bit?"

"Sure. See you later, babe," he says to the young lady. "I'm goin' to get my head shrunk up." She giggles as we head for the interview room.

I waste no time in getting to the point. "So, are you still having thoughts of killing yourself?"

"Oh, most definitely. I'm planning to go buy a gun and some bullets in the TL and get a crummy hotel room and blow my head off, once and for all." He says this with a half-crooked smile, his head cocked a bit to the side. "And I do know how to use a gun."

"As you've told me. And the nurse said you told her you've been hearing hallucinations, voices talking to you?"

"Oh, they're real bad. I'm hearin' them constantly, some dude's voice telling me to just go ahead and do it."

"How long have you heard voices?"

"They've been there constantly since I was a kid, as long as I can remember."

"And what age was that?"

"Oh, I think two, or maybe since I was a baby, one year old."

"Anything make the voices better?"

"Nope."

"And you've never told a doctor about this before?"

He smiles. "I never wanted anyone to think I was crazy."

All my red flags for malingering are flying now as if buffeted by a stiff breeze out of the northwest. Mr. Demerit's description of his auditory hallucinations screams, "Fake, fake, fake!" According to the forensic expert Dr. Phillip Resnick and others, genuine auditory hallucinations tend to be intermittent, are somewhat remediable by the sufferers, and very rarely start in childhood (and who can remember back to the second year of life?). Here's a guy who's allegedly been hearing voices all his life and yet has never found himself admitted to a psychiatric hospital or on psych meds. Here's a guy who has avoided arrest and could very well benefit from trying on a "psych jacket" for his future courtroom appearances.

The psych jacket can generally buy you time in a state hospital instead of the penitentiary; it's not necessarily a nice place, but it's a whole lot safer and more comfortable than the pen. It also might buy you Social Security disability benefits when you get out. (Though the feds have made it harder and harder for convicted felons to get benefits of any kind after their release.) Many criminals believe that donning a psych jacket gives them an excuse for criminal acts. Diminished capacity.

But as some psychiatric clinicians say, mental illness is no excuse for bad behavior. What this really means is that a whole lot of "bad behavior"—especially things like fraud, burglaries, and prevarications—is made up of volitional and intentional acts that often require a clear head and no small amount of premeditation and planning.

"I've been doing this work for more than ten years," I say. "I've seen thousands of patients, and, believe me, I know crazy."

"What are you trying to say, doctor?"

"Well, to put it bluntly, you don't seem crazy to me."

"You don't know what I'm goin' through."

"But even if you're not crazy—which is a good thing, by the way—it doesn't mean you don't have problems, like alcoholism, addiction, and being a criminal."

"So you're not gonna help me?"

"I never said I didn't think you needed help. You most certainly do. I'm just tryin' to figure this thing out."

"I appreciate that."

"A psych givin' you a sorta-clean bill of mental health is a very good thing."

"I see what you're sayin'."

"But I do notice that you seem a lot different this morning than yesterday."

"Yeah, man, I was still high last night."

"You seem to be in pretty good spirits today, though."

"Tears of a clown, doc, tears of a clown."

"What do you mean?"

"Well, I'm just trying to keep a happy face on things."

"What's been goin' on?"

"Well, I have a court date next week. And I might be looking at some heavy time."

"What are the charges?"

"Well, a lot of them, I'm afraid. Possession with intent to sell. Strong-armed robbery. Felony domestic violence."

"And how is it that the police didn't arrest you yesterday instead of bringing you here?"

"I guess you'd have to ask them. Less paperwork? I dunno."

"Okay, Rick, I need to give this some thought before I make a decision."

"You mean, you might not admit me? Doc, I need to be in the hospital."

"I'll check back with you in a little bit."

I return to the staff room to find the evaluating nurse. "Well, what do you think, doctor?" she asks.

"He seems pretty antisocial to me," I say. "He does state what sounds like a pretty lethal suicide plan. But nothing else adds up. The way he describes his voices, the little green men, the insistence on being admitted, the lack of an Axis I disorder other than substance abuse."

"And don't forget the secondary gain, Paul. An upcoming court date, lack of a psychiatric history, history of incarceration."

"Yeah, let's give him the boot. I hate to do it, but I don't think we have a choice."

"I'll call for a police escort out of the hospital."

"Yeah, a show of force. I think that's the only way he'll leave. I do hate to do it this way, but we're going to have to."

Mr. Demerit quietly packs his things with two men in blue standing by. I assume he has been shown the door out of multiple other venues. He doesn't say a word as he walks next to the men in blue out of the dayroom, except to his new girlfriend. "Bye, babe. Hope to see you out on the streets."

. . .

My evaluation of Rick Demerit came just a few years after I finished my residency. In those days I still routinely discharged patients I believed were malingering. I almost relished figuratively kicking patients like him to the curb.

I was 99 percent sure that Rick Demerit wouldn't kill himself. But was there something I could have offered him to help him change? I began to doubt that when I discovered that he didn't feel he had an alcohol or drug problem. Nor, in his estimation, did he have a problem with his temper. If he beat somebody, he said, it was only because they deserved it. Now, that's antisocial.

SEVEN

THE CLAIRVOYANT

Whose Life Is It Anyway?

"That was a profoundly decent thing to do," said my psychiatrist. I had just finished telling him about my meeting with the father of a young man, a one-visit patient now deceased, whom I had discharged from psych emergency only to have him commit suicide three days later by hanging.

I thought I detected soft tears in his eyes as he said this, but I couldn't be sure. Sometimes decency is all anyone has to offer to a grieving person. Yes, I could give myself credit for that. But one cannot undo what's been done—a man, a father like me, had not only lost his son; he'd lost his son to suicide, a supposedly preventable death.

I met with the young man's father for about half an hour outside the hospital, on a bench, under a warm spring sun. I did not hold back. I only vaguely considered the medicolegal consequences. I was guided by my conscience and my wish to provide comfort. "In retrospect, I wish I had made a different decision," I told him. "I wish I would have put him in the hospital, but I can't go back in time. I used my best judgment at the time. I'm sorry."

. . .

On the day in question, I read through the patient's paperwork—
the medical clearance, the paramedics' notes, the psychiatric
hold written by the police—before seeing him. It says that the
young man's father had called 911 at about two in the morning.
He had reported that his son had taken an overdose of ibuprofen while intoxicated. Most of the one hundred pills—in a bottle
previously full of two-hundred-milligram ibuprofen tablets—
were gone.

When police and paramedics had arrived on the scene, Will
O'Brien was difficult to rouse. The police officers placed him
on a seventy-two-hour involuntary psychiatric hold, and the
paramedics transported him to SFGH's Emergency Department. He was medically evaluated, given charcoal via a naso-
gastric tube, and then observed and monitored for several
hours before being transferred to the Psychiatric Emergency
Service on the basis of the "danger to self" criteria of the 5150
law.

Will O'Brien arrives in psych emergency on a Saturday
morning, and I evaluate him early that afternoon. My contact
with him begins when I go find him in the dayroom. He looks
even younger than his stated age of twenty. He sports a peach-
fuzz beard; probably he needs to shave no more than once a
week. Activated charcoal still ringing his lips, Will appears
downcast and says nothing.

This afternoon in the dayroom, a young woman picks at scabs
on her forearms, moaning, gently banging her head against the
wall, probably in response to traumatic memories or hallucinations. A very thin, wound-up little old lady paces back and forth,
singing old Broadway tunes repetitively, loudly, and off-key.

Two young men, clearly county jail graduates, yell at each other, threatening to punch each other's lights out: "Who *you* callin' *dog,* dog?" A middle-aged man puts his hand down his pajama bottoms and rolls his eyes. Instead of being alarmed by all the seriously disturbed patients surrounding him, Will doesn't even seem to notice them.

Will follows me into the interview room and sits down. The sun slices in through a high Plexiglas window. I need to move every few minutes to avoid getting blinded. Will sits with his back to the wall, his shoulders hunched, his posture slumped. He stares at a point between his feet and mine.

"Hi, Will, my name is Dr. Linde. I am one of the psychiatrists working here today. As you probably know, you are here on a 5150 hold, which means you can be held for up to seventy-two hours for a psychiatric evaluation. I can drop the hold and let you go sooner, or I may decide to continue it and make arrangements for you to be hospitalized."

He does not stir.

"The hold was placed by the police who responded to your father's call. I've read the notes from the paramedics and the ER, so I know a little bit about your situation. So, what's been happening in your life recently?" This is my version of the medical classic "So, what seems to be the problem?"

The young Mr. O'Brien sits there, providing no eye contact. I wait for a full minute at least. A more workmanlike approach is in order. "Did you take an overdose of ibuprofen, as the 5150 and the ER notes would indicate?"

"Yes."

"How many did you take?"

"I don't know."

"Could you make a guess? Was it just a few? Half a bottle?"

"A handful."

"What did you think would happen after you took the pills?"

Will pauses for nearly half a minute. "I don't know. I was drunk at the time."

"How much had you had to drink?"

"Well, a couple pints of Guinness, that's all. Out with the boys." I mentally note this as a serious underestimation, since I know his blood alcohol level in the ER had registered 170, and you can't get there with two pints.

"Do you remember taking the pills?" I think he may have been in an alcohol-induced amnestic state, informally called an alcoholic blackout, which implies a sort of dreamlike state in which one is still more or less functioning but of which one would have no recollection the morning after.

A pause. "Yes."

"What were you thinking about when you took the pills?" I ask, taking a slightly different tack to get at his state of mind.

"Nothing."

I wait, again nearly a minute, to see if he can, or will, add anything else. He remains silent. I understand his one-word response to this open-ended question as a sign that I need to keep making yes-or-no queries. This is less than optimal, but in this business you often have to take what you get.

"Have you ever attempted suicide before?"

"No."

"When you took the overdose, what were your intentions?"

"What do you mean?"

"What did you intend to happen?"

A long pause. "Well, just to go to sleep, I guess."

"Were you intending to die?"

"Maybe."

"Have you been thinking about wishing you were dead?"

"Yes."

"Have you been thinking about ways to kill yourself?"

"No."

"Do you or your dad have a gun at home?"

"No."

"Did you think you would die when you took the overdose?"

"I thought it might have been enough, but I wasn't sure."

I haven't entirely given up on the open-ended questions, and I bring them back into the mix now and then. "How do you feel about being alive now?" I've always found this question to be useful. I mean, "Here you are, you're alive. You didn't die."

Will O'Brien takes his time. He chokes up a bit and falters. His speech thickens. "Well, I wish I wasn't here."

"I see. Does that mean here in psych emergency, or here still on planet Earth?"

"Well, both, I guess."

I wait.

"It's my girlfriend," he says, swallowing. "She's breaking up with me."

"How long have you been together?"

"Two years."

"Was the breakup your idea or hers?"

"It wasn't mine," snarls Will, the first rise I'd seen out of him.

"When did she tell you she wanted to break up?"

"This past week."

"Did she tell you in person?"

"No, that's part of the problem. She's overseas. And I'm stuck here working and going to school. I'm afraid she's seeing different guys. She says she's not, but . . ." His voice trails off. "She says she loves me, but . . ." His speech halts again, but tears do not fall. If anything, his visage tightens. "But, but . . . but she feels like she's too young to get married. That she wants to date other guys before she settles down."

"How old is she?"

"Nineteen. I called her last night, before I took the overdose, to tell her I loved her."

"Were you calling to say good-bye?"

"No, not at all. I was calling to see if she'd reconsider. To let her know that I really love her, that this is no little-kid love. This is the real thing. Once in a lifetime. I told her that I can't imagine myself with anybody else."

"What did she say?"

He looks at the floor, holding his breath before exhaling loudly, trying to hold back tears. I sit quietly, expectantly. He doesn't cry. "She said . . ." He gulps and whispers his answer. "She said she didn't know for sure if I was the one. She said she loved me but she needed more time."

Recognizing the bittersweet punch of her statement, I exhale loudly, shake my head, and look down, pausing. "Boy, that's a tough one. How did you feel when she said that?"

"I felt determined," he says, his lip curling. "I'm sure she'll come back to me."

"Did you feel anything else?"

"No, just determined."

"Not sad?" I ask. "Not angry?"

Puzzled, he looks at me. "Sure, of course," he says. "But she *will* come back to me."

"For your sake, I hope so," I say. "It sounds like losing her could be a crushing blow."

"Yeah." He looks resigned.

I wait a bit. "What do you hope for in the future?"

"Other than marrying my girlfriend and starting a family?"

"Yes."

"Going back to school. Starting a business. I need to have a way to support her."

"Sure," I say. "Listen, Will, I need to give this situation some thought. On the face of it, it's a pretty serious suicide attempt, and I may need to put you in the hospital, on a psychiatric ward, to keep you from hurting yourself. But on the other hand, I'd rather not subject you to all of this," I say, gesturing in the direction of the dayroom, "any longer than absolutely necessary." In addition to the young woman, the elderly lady, the two young thugs, and the onanistic man, there is now a psychotic young Chinese man who intrudes on other patients, exposing his privates, speaking gibberish. Though he is a native speaker of Mandarin, his thought process reveals itself as nonsensical, even when he is interviewed later with the help of a fully bilingual interpreter. Of course, the staff and I try to intervene in situations like these—whether it involves putting patients in seclusion rooms, if available, or giving them extra medications or just telling them to stop engaging in their disruptive behaviors.

Will is a typical middle-class kid. He's never seen the inside of a place like this before. I find myself identifying with him—strongly. I can feel the pain of his breakup. Like anyone else, I had been jilted more than a few times as a teenager and young adult. I feel sorry for him.

"I may have to put you in the hospital to keep you safe, and start some treatment for depression. But if I don't have to, I won't. I'd like to speak with your father alone for a bit. Is that okay?"

"Sure."

"Then we'll meet together to come up with a plan."

. . .

Just as no two people are exactly alike, no two suicides are exactly the same. For some, it is a daring recreational maneuver that goes a little too far, often in the setting of drunkenness or a drug high. Momentary desperation impels others to jump off a cliff, a building, or a bridge or in front of an oncoming train or bus. If one is faced with a lethal opportunity in the here and now, death can be achieved impulsively, courtesy of an instantaneous decision. Once you've jumped over the four-foot railing of the Golden Gate Bridge and are hurtling downward, there's no turning back.

For many others, those who premeditate their demise, suicide can take weeks of planning and scheming: researching methods in books or on the Internet; buying a gun, learning how to shoot it, and obtaining ammunition; squirreling away enough pills; or sharpening a big knife, getting up the nerve to slice an artery, and making yourself scarce enough so as not to be discovered after the proximal deed is done, concealing your intent.

Psychologist Kay Redfield Jamison, in her memoir *An Unquiet Mind,* vividly describes her suffering, her recurrent thoughts of death, and the forethought that can go into a suicide attempt:

> From the time I woke up in the morning until the time I went to bed at night, I was unbearably miserable and seemingly

incapable of any kind of joy or enthusiasm. Everything—every thought, word, movement—was an effort. Everything that was once sparkling now was flat. I seemed to myself to be dull, boring, inadequate, thick brained, unlit, unresponsive, chill skinned, bloodless, and sparrow drab. . . .

The morbidity of my mind was astonishing: Death and its kin were constant companions. . . .

At one point I bought a gun, but, in a transient wave of rational thought, I told my psychiatrist; reluctantly, I got rid of it. Then for many months I went to the eighth floor of the stairwell of the UCLA hospital and, repeatedly, only just resisted throwing myself off the ledge. . . . The thought that my family would have to identify the fallen and fractured me made that ultimately not an acceptable method. . . .

I decided to take a massive overdose. . . . It was not a pleasant way not to commit suicide[,] . . . in and out of a coma for several days, which, given the circumstances, was probably just as well.[1]

For any psychiatrist, deciding whether to hospitalize a suicidal person is a delicate judgment call. The truth is that I can keep you alive by putting you in the hospital (even though a small subset of patients commits suicide on the psych ward), but after discharge, who knows? Unfortunately, no one, including psychiatrists, can accurately predict suicidal or homicidal behavior. Maybe I can project out a few hours after discharge, but after that it's hard to say. In one's life, there are too many variables, too many things that can go wrong. Relationships splinter; children get sick; people get fired; friends split; arguments happen; financial problems loom. It is just as important, if not more essential, to consider the factors that mitigate the risk:

The Clairvoyant / 149

Feeling prohibited from completing suicide by either
strongly held religious beliefs or not wanting to traumatize
the would-be survivors.

Holding on to hope for the future—plans for a significant
relationship, a career, having children, or other future-ori-
ented goals.

Expressing ambivalence about dying, and being able to
accentuate and highlight the positives, the reasons for living.
A lack of ambivalence, with an attendant determination to
die, is a serious risk factor.

Having a strong and available support system is key.
Conversely, the experiences of shame, secrecy, social isolation, and not wanting to burden or burn out friends or
family members all increase the risk of suicide.

Psychiatrists are held to a legal standard in evaluating the
risk, whether acute or chronic, of suicide, and in documenting
the factors that increase or mitigate the risk. A judge or jury will
not (or at least shouldn't) hold psychiatrists to a higher standard,
one that would require the otherworldly skill of clairvoyance.

Despite the unpredictability of suicide, it is my responsibility
to do the best I can, to apply my best professional judgment in
deciding who needs admission and who is okay to leave. But I
often let patients in on the dilemma. My stance is: "Hey, it's your
life, it's your body, it's your mind, so I'm going tell you how I
make this decision. Really only you know, deep down, whether
you're going to go through with this suicide thing."

This approach does not work for every patient, and it doesn't
work for many psychiatrists, but it's my preferred way of doing

business. Ultimately there is no small amount of free will involved in the decision to take one's own life. Sure, there are treatable problems that need to be aggressively addressed, but at the end of the day it's one's own call.

I might say, "In the long run, I can't keep you from killing yourself. If you want to do it badly enough, then you'll find a way. I can't keep you locked up forever. There will come a day in the not-so-distant future when you'll be out on your own. I'm here to help you find reasons for sticking around, for going on, to help you find meaning in life or a sense of purpose or community—some reason, any reason, for you to not kill yourself."

In these situations, it is essential to find the ambivalence and explore it. "What is it that you want to live for? What gives you hope? What will you miss if you're gone? Who will miss you?" I remind them that their decisions and actions can set in motion consequences that are complex and often unintended.

For the average person, it may seem hard to believe that many people keep suicide on their list of possible coping strategies should their pain become too great. I've talked to hundreds of people who would never consider removing suicide from their list of options. For many of them, paradoxically, keeping it on the list is the one thing that prevents them from actually doing it. Anita Darcel Taylor, a writer who suffers from bipolar disorder, also known as manic-depressive illness, puts it this way:

> At its worst, manic depression is hell, and each time I cycle through an episode, a few more of life's pleasures are stripped away. One should be forced to pass through hell once. Twice maximum. At 47, I have been to its depth a definitive six times.
>
> I have no grand wish for death. I do not view suicide as a desire to end life or a dramatic way to go down in flames. Rather,

it is a tool in my possession—the only one, really—that offers a permanent end to my pain. When I have lost enough of myself to this disease as to become unrecognizable even to me, I will stop. I will go no further. That, I tell myself, is my earned choice.[2]

To patients like Ms. Taylor, I often say something like this: "I understand you're not likely to take suicide off your list, but I'd like you to push it from second or third place back down to seventh or eighth or, better yet, fifteenth."

. . .

By now Will's father has arrived at the psych ER. I sit down with him to gain his perspective. Matthew O'Brien, in his mid-forties, is tan and fit, with tousled brown hair graying at the sideburns. He smiles easily, genuinely. He speaks softly, wringing his callused hands as he talks. "Have you heard Will talk at all about suicide or even wishing that he were dead?" I start.

"No. It all came as a shock to me. I mean, I could see that he was down. I knew that his girlfriend had broken up with him on the phone, a transatlantic call, and that that had sent him into a slump. He was mopey, not saying much, sleeping in. He started to drink more when he went out with his friends. I figured he'd be okay. Oh, I know it hurts going through a breakup. I'm afraid I remember the feeling all too well, but after a week or two you snap out of it. You start thinking about other girls. You go out with your buddies.

"The two of them were just too close. They were already acting like an old married couple at the age of nineteen. They hardly even went out on dates anymore—they'd just sit at home and watch videos. I encouraged him to go out with his friends once in a while, but he even stopped doing that. He was crazy in love with her, and she seemed to like looking after him. He was very jealous, very possessive. He didn't like the fact that other guys were noticing her when she went to school. She is an attractive young lady and very nice. She kept reassuring him that she wasn't interested in other guys, and that she loved him and would remain faithful to him, but he still worried about it."

"Has Will ever attempted suicide before?" I ask. "As far as you know."

"No, I'm pretty sure he hasn't."

"Has he ever been on psychiatric medications?"

"Not that I know of. I doubt it."

"Has he ever talked to a psychiatrist or to a therapist in the past?"

"No, but maybe he should have."

"Should have when?" I ask.

"Oh, after his mother died. He was nine years old at the time. We were separated and divorced by the time he was four, and he was living with her. Mary was killed in an auto accident, drunk driver. Just awful."

"Did Will have brothers or sisters from your marriage?"

"No, he was an only child. We had infertility problems," says Mr. O'Brien.

"Did you raise him after that?"

"No. I know it sounds bad, but I had moved away by then, and he was pretty well set in his school. Mary's parents lived in the area. They were young for their age, if you know what I mean, so they pretty much raised him. I saw him as often as I could, maybe twice a month, but I was busy working."

"How did the arrangement work out?"

"Pretty well. Will's grandparents were terrific people, and they really loved him and took good care of him."

"But still it's not the same as being raised by your parents," I say, almost reflexively. I don't say this to make Mr. O'Brien feel bad, but to make a mental note of just how traumatic his mother's death must have been for Will.

"Yes," he says. "And I almost forgot, he lost his grandmother to heart disease last year. He was very close to her, and she doted on him."

"Boy, that's a lot of losses to endure," I say. "And now another one with this breakup."

"After my marriage broke up, I went into a bit of a depression myself. I threw myself into my work, which helped the company do well financially but left me little time to spend with my son, who needed me after his mother died." Mr. O'Brien grows quiet.

"You obviously love your son," I say. "You did what you thought was best at the time."

"Maybe," he says. "I also started drinking a lot more to deal with the pain. Drinking on the job was not such a big deal back then. It was okay to have alcohol on your breath during the day, as long as you didn't seem too drunk or stupid or belligerent."

"Are you still drinking?" I ask.

"Oh, no, I gave that up about five years ago."

"Why then?"

"Well, I had just met my girlfriend, who is now my wife, and I had recently hit forty. She didn't like my drinking too much— she doesn't drink at all—and the hangovers were really getting to me, so I just quit."

"Did you go to AA?" I ask.

"Nah, I just quit on my own. It wasn't too hard. A lot of the guys on my crews had also quit, and my wife doesn't drink, of course."

"Do you have a family history of suicide? Uncles, aunts, cousins, grandparents?"

"No. Though several of my relatives have suffered problems with alcoholism and depression, none of 'em to the point of being in the hospital or anything like that."

"Are you and Will close?"

"We're very close now," says Mr. O'Brien. His eyes light up. His face brightens. "Every night we talk about things. He has told me a lot about his hurt feelings in this relationship. I've done my best to be supportive. But at a certain point it was clear to me that she wasn't going to come back to him. I felt he should move on. There's a lot of fish in the sea. I encouraged him to start dating girls here. He had some female friends, but no one that he ever dated. You know, he has plans for the future. He's talked to me about going to trade school, maybe helping me out in the business or getting his own one going."

"So, who else is in your family?" I ask. "Who does Will live with?"

"Well, with me and my wife. We've been together for almost six years, married for four. And with my younger son, Peter, who is almost three years old."

"You sound like a busy man. How does your wife treat Will?"

"Like her own. She's only about twelve years older than Will, so maybe he feels more like she's an aunt or a big sister to him. My wife and Will talk all the time. It seems to be a very comfortable relationship."

"And how about Will and son number two?"

"Oh, he's crazy about him. He's always playing with him, wrestling with him on the floor, buying him little toys."

"That's nice," I say.

"Come to think of it, lately, it's about the only time I see Will smile. Yeah. I guess I'm trying to make up for lost time." Mr. O'Brien hangs his head and pauses here a bit. "I still feel bad I wasn't really there for him during his teenage years. I mean, he was well taken care of by his grandparents. He didn't lack for nothin' materially, but, it's just that . . ."

"Just what?" I ask.

"It's just that Will became such a loner, which was not at all what he was like when he was younger. His grades suffered, he used to be a straight-A student. But I was so lost in my own grief, my work, my drinking, that I didn't apply myself to helping him."

We trade stories about being middle-aged fathers to preschoolers. It is obvious that Mr. O'Brien loves Will with all his heart. I think he also wants to take the pain away, to make things all better. We share that wish. It's a dangerous identification, as it can bring out the rose-colored glasses.

. . .

Before I met with Will and his father together, I had not made up my mind about whether to hospitalize him. Given my interaction with Matthew O'Brien, I was leaning toward letting Will go. After all, it would mean releasing Will to a loving home where two adults who cared about him could keep an eye on him. And it would entail starting Will on an antidepressant medication and linking him with our short-term case management team so he could be seen early the following week.

I so wanted to believe that everything would be all right—
that Will would be okay and get on with his life and overcome
his substantial losses. Will seemed fortunate to have a father
who was so emotionally healthy, supportive, and available. In
talking to Matthew O'Brien, I saw a father who was vastly
"new and improved"—ready to make up for lost time to the
best of his ability.

I am a father as well, and I saw Mr. O'Brien as one of the good
guys. I thought, "This is a guy who can handle it, who will save
his son because of his essential goodness and generosity." Maybe
it was because I had to deal with so many damaged people in the
hospital environment that Mr. O'Brien seemed superlative in
comparison. From a more objective perspective, one could point
to substantial risk factors that could predispose Will to attempt
suicide again, including his major depression, his having just
attempted a moderately lethal overdose, his ongoing feelings of
emotional loss and abandonment made acute by his breakup
with his girlfriend, and his ambivalence about still being alive.

In retrospect, I wish I had made a different decision. Things
are always clearer when viewed through the "retrospectoscope."
And though predicting suicide is still very challenging, more
recent thinking has clarified the process to some extent. In the
late 1990s, the psychiatrist Shawn Christopher Shea identified
and put into practice a systematic approach to suicide risk assessment. The Chronological Assessment of Suicide Events, a.k.a.
the CASE approach, can be understood as a guideline for interviewing a suicidal patient and then assessing his or her suicidal
risk.[3] Dr. Shea outlines four separate variables, four different
regions for exploration, organized by chronology, to consider in
making a comprehensive risk assessment.

Region 1 exploration addresses suicide events. In plain terms, this means an interviewer tries to obtain the particulars of the clinical story predating the patient's arrival. Suicidal thoughts and behavior cover a wide spectrum. These range from expressing a passive wish to die (such as by falling asleep tonight and never waking up), to actively planning and intending suicide by lethal means, to having just made a serious attempt at suicide.

The events of interest to the interviewer include the circumstances prior to a patient's arrival to psych emergency—the wheres, whens, whats, whys, and hows of method, premeditation, potential lethality, covertness, alcohol or drug use, specific life stressors and losses, and other variables. The psychiatrist uses techniques when interviewing that are similar to those of an adept news reporter.[4]

Region 2 exploration focuses on recent suicidal events. This involves looking at the two months prior to the interview and especially examining the types and intensities of suicidal thoughts and actions.[5] This line of investigation requires the interviewer to be sophisticated not only in gathering facts but also in identifying and exploring a person's psychological responses to stresses and losses in the previous two months. According to Shea, this might be the most important area of inquiry.

Region 3 exploration covers past suicidal events, specifically those occurring more than two months prior to the current assessment, and chronicling patterns of suicidal thoughts and behaviors. This is an investigation into a person's psychiatric history—the circumstances of past suicidal thoughts and, more important, suicide attempts. In sum, past behavior can at least help foretell future behavior.[6]

Region 4 is the person's state of mind while being evaluated. Pertinent questions here include: Are you still suicidal? How do you feel about being alive? If you're not suicidal now, what's changed?[7]

My knowledge of Shea's approach was fuzzy at the time that I assessed Will O'Brien—certainly much fuzzier than it is now, a decade later. While mental health professionals have been aware of these suicide risk factors for several years, credit is due Shea for creating a framework that makes the assessment of suicide risk more systematic. Nonetheless, it is difficult to disregard the subjective gut feelings inherent to this kind of psychiatric evaluation. Sometimes these instincts point you toward a better decision, and at other times, well, the opposite is true. This is where I stumbled with Will O'Brien.

. . .

As I sit down with Matthew and Will O'Brien in the interview room, not having fully made up my mind but leaning toward letting Will go, I try to instill hope in the downcast young man. "I know what it's like to get dumped. It sucks. It hurts. And it's gonna hurt for a while. But the clouds will eventually clear, and you'll find someone else you will love and who will love you even more."

My identifying with him, a sincere attempt at empathy, apparently leads me to inappropriately normalize his condition. It apparently blinds me to the seriousness of his depression and his suicide attempt. I am pulling for him, wanting not only to spare him the experience of a *Cuckoo's Nest* but also to see him off to a good life. "Hey, you're young, you're a good-looking guy. There's lots of other fish in the sea; you've just got to get out there. You've got a long life ahead of you." Will sits there as his father nods his head and smiles, an indication that he's been down this road with Will himself. "I can tell your father loves you very much and wants what's best for you. Still, we need to decide whether or not it would make sense for you to go into the hospital. What do you think?"

Will sits there, a deer in the headlights. Finally, he says, "Well, if it was up to me, I'd rather not."

Respect for patient autonomy is an ethical pillar of clinical medicine and psychiatry. Though it's my responsibility to make an informed decision, to try to protect patients, I must also take into account the wishes of the patient. "Will, I've had a chance to think about things," I tell him. "I think you're suffering from a major depression. It's something that's treatable, and the vast majority of people with it do get better with treatment. A full recovery can take two or three months, but if we get going with therapy and medications, we can get you feeling better in the first week or two. Do you think you're at risk to kill yourself if you leave the hospital?" I ask.

A hesitation. "No. I don't want to go through anything like this again."

On the face of it, the statement implies that the experience of having his stomach pumped was aversive enough that Will doesn't want to repeat it. But, if one looks more deeply, it can be construed as ominous: "Well, if I do successfully kill myself, I won't be coming through this hospital again, and I won't ever have to have my stomach pumped again."

"What would you do if, either later tonight or tomorrow morning, you felt intensely suicidal?" I ask.

Without hesitating, Will says, "I'd tell my dad."

Matthew O'Brien breathes out audibly—an apparent sigh of relief.

After a discussion of risks and benefits, Will agrees to begin taking Prozac. He also agrees to meet with one of our short-term crisis case managers. I give him the phone number, and I leave a message for the crisis team. I know he can see one of their psychiatrists within a week to assess the early effects of the medication. The availability of that referral and his acceptance of it are both good signs.

I decide to let Will have his freedom. I trust him to come back for more treatment, but more important, I trust him to carry on, to persevere.

"Can you promise me that you won't do anything to hurt yourself?'

"Yes."

"Can you promise me that you will talk to somebody if you're feeling suicidal, instead of doing something to hurt yourself?"

"Yes."

For many years, this "no-harm contract," or safety plan, was invoked to indemnify the psychiatrist in case of a completed suicide. But as multiple studies have shown, the beloved no-harm contract is not worth a hill of beans. For many patients, it does provide a measure of safety and support, a tangible remembrance that others are now aware of their suicidal thoughts and impulses. But for others, for those who've more or less decided on suicide as a final solution, it is an empty promise meant to falsely reassure. Will, however, signaled to me that he was willing to try taking an antidepressant medication, and that he would follow up with a counselor.

"I'll make certain he makes his appointment and also keep an eye on him," says Will's father.

"I will let you go," I say.

Will seems genuinely pleased to be able to leave the hospital. His father seems worn out but is able to manage a smile to go with his firm handshake.

During the rest of the shift, after I discharge Will, I become immersed in the never-ending human suffering, crisis after crisis, some bizarre, that continues to stream in our doors on that busy Saturday. In the rush of new problems to address, I soon forget about Will. I do not lose sleep over the case that night. It's the kind of decision I have to make at least two or three times a week.

No one but God can truly see inside the human psyche, spirit, or soul. No one can foretell the future. You do the best you can, and you move on. But the degree of effort and the quality of the outcome are not necessarily proportional.

. . .

Three days later, I get a message to phone the hospital's risk manager. Never a good sign.

"Dr. Linde?" the voice on the other end of the line asks. "This is Mr. Downing from Risk Management. I've got some bad news for you."

"Yes," I say. "I'm listening."

"Will O'Brien was found dead at his father's home this morning. All signs point to a suicide. He hanged himself." When Will said that he could not live without his girlfriend, he must have meant it literally.

Mr. Downing speaks for another three or four minutes, but I hear little of it. I numb out for a while. I do tune back in when he speaks to me about scheduling an "M and M" with me. I wish "M and M" stood only for candy. It also stands for the morbidity and mortality conference, which is held in a hospital after a bad outcome, presumably to learn from a mistake, to do some fact-finding, and as a defensive maneuver from a legal perspective.

My first defense is denial. But before long, my tack is simply to blame myself. What had I done? Or not done? I go round and round then, a ball of confusion. I, of course, talk to my therapist about it. I feel like I deflect the pain. I nullify the pain. I do not want to take it on. I do take it on. It feels personal. I can relate. I want to make it all better. I want to run from it. I still want to believe that everything will turn out all right.

Then I move into the what-if stage, the wish to undo. Would I have saved his life by admitting him to the hospital? Well, for at least the time he was in the hospital. Unless he pulled a fast one and killed himself on the psych ward, I would have saved his life for the amount of time he spent in the ward under obser-vation. At a minimum I could have forestalled his death. Yes, maybe it was inevitable, but I'd like a chance for a do-over.

Then I veer toward rationalization by saying, "Hey, suicide happens, it could happen to anyone," which is true, of course. My thinking at the time goes something like this: A psychiatrist working in the emergency service of a busy county hospital works with the sickest of the sick, all of whom pose a greater risk of completing suicide than the fictional "average" person. The misery quotient in psych emergency is high. The afflictions I see are some of humanity's greatest and most tragic: AIDS, homelessness, poverty, alcoholism, addiction, major depression, chronic pain, bipolar disorder, schizophrenia, the emotional effects of torture, social isolation, the aftermath of fresh and major losses, and the experience of being terminally ill. And of course, added to the list of those who pose a greater risk are those who have just attempted suicide and those who have a history of attempting suicide. But my rationalization, though it works pretty well to distance myself from this terrible tragedy, doesn't work for long.

The defenses of denial, undoing, and rationalization fail to make me feel much better. I need to feel the grief, feel the loss, and tolerate it to begin to heal. Will O'Brien should have been just another young man with a future full of love and work and heartbreak and joy, just like anyone else at the age of twenty. And I could have prevented his exit from this material world. Matthew O'Brien shouldn't have been deprived of the chance to see his son grow, change, and develop into an adult with hopes and dreams.

When I speak with Matthew O'Brien on the phone a few days after Will's suicide, I am relieved that he agrees to meet with me face-to-face to talk more about Will's death. At first, I am extremely nervous about meeting with Mr. O'Brien. But doing so seems like the right thing to do. I am genuinely sad about his loss and wish I had made a different decision. What helps me heal most is the forgiveness he offers me in our brief meeting on the bench outside after Will's death. It is clear to me that his decency clears the way for his forgiveness.

. . .

The most important lesson I learned from the experience was this: Be very aware of the risks of overidentifying with a patient. It's another spin on the old line "If it feels so right, how can it go so wrong?" Unfortunately, although an emotional identification with patients can lead one to an empathic and nuanced response in the moment, it can also blind one to an increased risk in decision making. The identification can literally cloud one's judgment.

I did become clinically conservative for at least several months after Will's death, deciding to hospitalize a great majority of suicidal patients that I came across. Over time, that extra caution gave way to a more balanced and considered judgment. A few good things came out of the experience:

I believe I became more seasoned and adept at making suicide risk assessments. Specifically, I'm now less likely to be blinded by overly identifying with my patients. And I'm more attuned to recognizing the vulnerability of feeling abandoned and experiencing recent, major losses, which in Will's case were part of a lifetime of losses.

Matthew O'Brien became actively involved in working with other survivors of suicide. He attended meetings of groups that he found helpful, and he decided he would get some extra training and learn how to facilitate those groups.

Unfortunately, none of these things could change what happened. Or bring Will O'Brien back to life.

EIGHT

THE SPEED COP

Talking to Tina

In psych emergency, sometimes it seems like everyone is on speed. It's like this: A guy comes in all wild-eyed and crazy. Often he's been violent in the community and sometimes in the hospital. He steadfastly denies using crystal methamphetamine. Maybe he suffers from bipolar disorder, also called manic-depressive illness, and he's gotten manic since he stopped taking his lithium. Maybe, but it sure looks like meth behavior, and frankly, much of the psychotic and violent behavior around these parts is assumed to be driven by meth intoxication until proven otherwise. Meth or mania, mania or meth. It's easy to get fooled.

Often we'll get a call from a patient's parent or his psychiatrist and find out that indeed the guy does have bipolar disorder and doesn't use drugs. The conversation might go something like this: "No, he doesn't use drugs. I know, doctor, I know, it sure does look like drugs, but he really doesn't use drugs, and he's gone off his psych meds again. Usually does this time of year, and, no, he doesn't use drugs—he's a health nut. No alcohol, no cigarettes, not even coffee."

We still might be skeptical. But when we get back a clean urine toxicological screen from the lab, that pretty much seals the deal—it's plain old mania. In psych emergency, we understand this situation in blunt terms: to be that psychotic without being on drugs indicates a severe psychiatric illness.

It may seem strange to wish that a urine tox screen will be positive for cocaine or methamphetamine. But if the use of a stimulant is the sole cause of a person's behavioral disturbance, it's good news because those effects generally wear off within hours or days. By contrast, a severe manic episode can last for weeks, even with aggressive pharmacologic treatment.

Addiction to stimulants can be "cured" if one ceases to use the drugs for good. In most cases, bipolar disorder can only be managed, not wiped out. Some manic-depressive patients make matters worse by abusing alcohol or drugs.

Taking meth while manic is like Han Solo kicking the *Millennium Falcon* into hyperdrive—one becomes the fastest object in the vicinity. And, like the Grateful Dead song says: "Too much of everything is just enough. . . . I need a miracle every day."[1] Using methamphetamine, especially when you inject it intravenously or smoke it, can feel like a miracle, I'm afraid.

. . .

The first time I see Mark Hill in the outpatient methamphetamine addiction clinic, he looks pretty good. He is calm, polite, articulate, soft spoken, and dressed in worn but clean clothes. He seems at least "ten degrees off," with some residual grandiosity and paranoia, but not too bad for a guy who has been shooting crystal meth into his veins for the last twenty years.

He tells me about a lingering, smoldering depression dating back to his childhood. I perform due diligence and elicit enough information to readily identify criteria of a clinical or major depression. He tells me he hasn't used in ten days—but only because his "good connection" of four years has been rolled up by the SFPD.

Mr. Hill doesn't trust the stuff he gets from other dealers, so he decides to give it a rest for the time being. He thinks he can kick speed this time because his stellar connection is likely to do more than a little jail time this go-round. I am naively optimistic that this might actually be true.

"I've really had it. I can't go on like this. This shit is tearing me up. My brain, my body. I gotta give it up or it'll kill me."

Mr. Hill is already being treated with a sedating antipsychotic medication, Seroquel, which if nothing else helps him sleep. He denies hearing hallucinations. I can't entirely discount his conspiracy theories concerning the government and police: the city of San Francisco has recently erected crime-monitoring video cameras atop poles in the more dangerous parts of the city, another manifestation of Big Brother. But what Mr. Hill thinks the government is doing with the videotapes sounds more elaborate than is likely true. His story and the detailed nature of his belief system make me suspect that he is suffering from paranoid ideas. I love that: I'm *suspicious* that Mr. Hill is suspicious. It makes me think of those now yellowing crime-fighting signs from ten or fifteen years earlier that say: Report suspicious people.

Suspicious people report suspicious people. Suspicious people report suspicious people report suspicious people.

Add paranoia, stir and repeat, stir and repeat, stir and repeat. Paranoia is a common complication of frequent, chronic intravenous methamphetamine use, which exactly fits Mark Hill's history.

I enjoy meeting Mr. Hill. I know helping him is going to be an uphill battle, but we have a good beginning here. I start him on an antidepressant medication. I'm hoping this might help him stop or at least cut down on his use of meth, though the research literature is mixed on this point. I make a follow-up appointment in two weeks and send him on his way.

. . .

The slang term *speed* refers both to the substance and the effect of illicit methamphetamines, which can be used in several different ways—most commonly by swallowing, snorting, smoking, or intravenous injection. Dextroamphetamine, with its nearly identical chemical structure, is a pharmaceutical sibling of methamphetamine. D-amphetamine is the active ingredient of the name-brand legal prescription stimulants Dexedrine and Adderall. Methylphenidate, pharmacologically a first cousin of methamphetamine, is the active ingredient of Ritalin. These legal stimulants are the mainstay of treatment for attention-deficit/hyperactivity disorder (ADHD)—which has been described in both children and adults—and sometimes are used as adjunctive medications for treatment-resistant major depression. Their addiction potential is much less than that of methamphetamine, not because of their slight chemical difference, but because of how they are introduced into the body.

After swallowing, pills are absorbed slowly in the stomach and small intestine. The ingested amphetamine undergoes metabolism by the liver and then gets distributed throughout the body via the circulatory system. When injected, smoked, or snorted, the stuff goes straight to your head, specifically your brain, within seconds or minutes. That's where the euphoric rush is generated: the faster and more intense the rush, the sooner and deeper the addiction.

Nicolas Rasmussen provides a fascinating history of amphetamine prescribing and marketing in America's twentieth century.[2] Amphetamines were originally synthesized in 1929 by Gordon Alles and initially tested as an inhaled treatment for asthma. Amphetamine was marketed as Benzedrine by the then pharmaceutical giant Smith, Kline and French and tried with varying success as a treatment for narcolepsy, low blood pressure, allergies, premenstrual syndrome, and cardiac disease.

Sometimes referred to as a "drug looking for a disease," amphetamine sulfate, in the form of Benzedrine tablets, received FDA approval in 1939 for the treatment of "neurotic depression." It was later marketed aggressively as a weight-loss agent because of its property of appetite suppression.

In the 1940s and 1950s, stimulants were seen as a conduit to lowering inhibitions of psychotherapy patients recumbent on psychoanalytic couches. National psychiatric trade journals of the 1950s in fact tout amphetamines as an effective tool for overcoming "blocking" in the patient who is undergoing psychoanalysis. Ironically enough, this era's popular but illegal designer drugs—the old standbys LSD and Ecstasy (methylenedioxymethamphetamine, a.k.a. MDMA or X)—were originally hailed as tools for breakthroughs in psychotherapy as well. Other "club drugs," such as gamma hydroxybutyrate (GHB, or G), ketamine (special K), and phencyclidine (PCP or angel dust), were borrowed from the legitimate world of anesthesia.[3] It makes one wonder about the genesis of tomorrow's party drugs—in particular which compounds remain a twinkle in the eye of some mad genius or have already been manufactured by some anonymous designer chemist.

Crystal methamphetamine is the gold standard for illegal stimulants, making cocaine seems like child's play. When meth is ingested, snorted, smoked, shot intravenously, or squirted into the rectum ("a booty bump"), it causes one to experience an intense rush, reminiscent of the "fight, flee, or fuck" response, inducing increased energy, elevated mood, heightened awareness, and increased alertness. When this response goes overboard, one becomes saddled with anxiety, insomnia, irritability, palpitations, hypertension, tremors, restlessness, and potential psychotic symptoms—paranoia, voices, visions, and the sensation of bugs crawling over the body. But the Grail of meth use is the heightened interest in sex it induces, which goes through the roof. That's what keeps a lot of people coming back for more.

Crystal is a purer, higher-grade, more expensive form of methamphetamine in comparison to its impoverished cousin, crank, which is generally cut with other junk and usually only snorted. The appeal of crank, which comes in the form of a yellowish brown powder, is that twenty dollars can get you high for several hours—in contrast to crack cocaine, twenty dollars of which will buy you only about a half hour of fun.

Hardly anyone in San Francisco uses crank. It seems to be much more a rural phenomenon, the output of primitive meth labs throughout the United States. Plenty of folks in the city still smoke crack cocaine—not at the rate seen in the 1980s, of course. But among San Francisco's connoisseurs of stimulants, it's all about crystal, also called "Crissy" or "Tina." It's worth the extra money, or so I am told. The purest forms of crystal meth appear in the form of clear to white glass shards, or "crystals." These are generally crushed into a powder for smoking or snorting or dissolved in some liquid for swallowing, injecting, or booty bumping.[4]

Lower grades of crystal are often cut with god-knows-what—talcum, powdered sugar, laundry detergent, baking soda, flour, or acidic solvents. The injection of these substances can soon obliterate the antecubital vein, the one in the crook of your arm that can reach nearly the size of a garden hose in a healthy young man.

With months and months of escalating use, chasing the high, one's brain chemicals, particularly dopamine and norepinephrine, become depleted, causing a syndrome that looks indistinguishable from a major depressive episode. The acute version of this—when one becomes fatigued, drowsy, melancholic, irritable, anhedonic, maybe even suicidal—is what meth users refer to as "the crash," the inevitable withdrawal from a two- or three-day stimulant binge. The cruel irony here is that a lot of meth addicts start out using speed to self-medicate symptoms of depression. In the short run, meth is a bitchin' good antidepressant. In the long run, it's a supergnarly depressant. Much as an alcoholic will drink a hair-of-the-dog cocktail to soothe his hangover, the crashing meth user will do another line or take another shot to get "well"—to counteract the debilitating physical and emotional symptoms of the crash.

This pharmacological reality can propel one into a particularly vicious downward spiral of using meth in larger amounts and more frequently in order to treat what has become a deepening depression. More ominously, meth use, with its attendant sleep deprivation, can cause an acute case of psychotic agitation characterized by hallucinations, pressured speech, fidgeting, pacing, and feelings of persecution. These behavioral manifestations are accompanied by the most telltale signs of all—dilated pupils, rapid heart rate, high blood pressure, and sometimes a low-grade fever. We see this syndrome often in psych emergency—ergo our dilemma: is it meth or mania?

Long-term meth use can also cause a chronic psychosis similar to a mild case of schizophrenia. Its sufferers often experience difficult-to-treat sequelae of paranoia, poorly formed hallucinations, and general befuddlement. So you *can* actually blow your mind on drugs, especially with stimulants like methamphetamine and, to a lesser extent, hallucinogens like LSD.

. . .

On the day of Mark Hill's second visit to the meth clinic, he actually arrives early for his appointment. I'm able to see him early due to the cancellation of one of my previous appointments. He tells me he's homeless again—he is sure his predominantly Spanish-speaking peers in the shelter were "talking shit about me," so he felt he had to leave. "It's no big deal, doc. I'm usually homeless for more than half the month."

He has some papers for me to sign. He is extremely restless, shifting endlessly in his chair, standing up, sitting down again, rummaging in his pockets for forgotten receipts, foraging through a stack of crinkled papers, looking for a specific housing referral form, never finding it. I ask him not *if* he's used, but at what time he shot up. He tells me he slammed that morning, a couple hours earlier. I ask him if he thinks it affects him at all, in any way, hoping for him to put two and two together—to say, "Yes, yes, it makes me a disorganized and anxious scrambled rambler, unable to perform any meaningful task." But as he grinds his teeth and rotates his jaw and sweats and fidgets, he tells me with a straight face, looking right into my eyes, "No, no, the speed doesn't affect me at all."

I protest mildly. "Mark, you're a mess today. When I saw you last week, you were calm, you were thoughtful, you were articulate, you were organized. And today, well, you're a bit of a wreck."

"A wreck?" he fumes. He continues shifting and picking through his papers and coughing and clearing his throat. "Well, it's because I haven't had a place to stay. How do you think you'd act if you didn't have a place to stay?" Denial is a hallmark of addiction. How am I going to get this guy to stop if he doesn't even see it as a problem, even though he so obviously becomes transformed into a disorganized mess after injecting meth? But as I sit back and listen to Mr. Hill for the next half hour, I begin to see how the meth unlocks him, calms him, and even frees him.

Today Mr. Hill is nobody's scapegoat, a role he played—the humiliated one—in his family because his biological father was not the same one his three half siblings had. His biological father was a rat, abandoning Mr. Hill and his mother while she was pregnant with him. Mr. Hill became an emotional whipping boy and physical punching bag for the family. His mother and stepfather beat him regularly—that is, until he grew into a lanky thirteen-year-old who learned to fight back and do no small amount of damage. The Family Court labeled him as "an incorrigible."

As a result, Mr. Hill got farmed out to a juvenile delinquents' camp, where he stood as a man-child among boys. He was a tall thirteen-year-old surrounded by savvy and sadistic sixteen-year-olds. So he learned to fight even more. First he fought in self-defense, but eventually he became the best brawler, the king of his juvey camp by the time he turned fifteen. On his sixteenth birthday, the wise and omniscient Family Court declared him irredeemable, unacceptable even for juvey camp. A monster. A badass. He was found to be an emancipated minor and was more or less kicked out of the camp to fend for himself.

Mr. Hill migrated to San Francisco during the Summer of Love and became an ungainly urchin alcoholic, hanging with hippies and runaways, having his first sexual experiences with women. He experienced more injustice, so he drank and drank and drank and drank and drank until he discovered a better way to blot out his misery. Methamphetamines.

It was now the early 1970s, and hedonism was *en vogue*. He got a regular girlfriend, a meth addict, and learned to snort meth because it was easier, it was manageable, and he could stop anytime he wanted to, no problem, he was not an addict. How could he be an addict when it felt so good?

Friend to Harley riders and true Hell's Angels, Mr. Hill finds that it helps to have good connections when you're a hardcore dope fiend and a regular, good-paying customer. Money talks and bullshit walks. He is not a real criminal but a low-level runner and lookout. Not a full brother but a faithful, loyal associate and good customer. "I'm not a snitch. Snitches don't survive around here," he intones.

Mr. Hill created a reality because his real reality, his childhood, was too damaging and traumatic to be believed, like that of combat veterans who actually saw hell on earth. It's buried, but when it comes out, you can believe it. Only true worms make up stuff—and they are out there, but are few and far between.

He suffers expansively when he shoots methamphetamine into his veins. His brain stays a little wobbly and psychotic even when he's not under the influence. With meth, his *qi* flows until he is a larger-than-life, self-described "monster" who takes orders from no one, who plays by nobody's rules, who refuses to be yelled at.

He has found a unique way to manage his traumatic past. He is doing it his own way, which represents a type of freedom.

Psychiatrist and concentration camp survivor Viktor Frankl describes a universal truth in his book *Man's Search for Meaning:* "Everything can be taken from a man but one thing: the last of the human freedoms—to choose one's attitude in any given set of circumstances, to choose one's own way. . . . It is this spiritual freedom—which cannot be taken away—that makes life meaningful and purposeful."[5]

Though he's been using regularly, Mr. Hill tells me that lately he's been thinking about getting into a program. I tell him that, if this is true, he should come see me in psych emergency the next Wednesday—a day on which I might be able to find him a residential treatment bed. It's not too much of a long shot. I pride myself on my advocacy and my creativity in getting patients to the places and things they need most.

.   .   .

Meth users fall into three broad categories—those who self-medicate psychiatric symptoms, those who use speed to increase work productivity, and those who use it to enhance sex. Many users take meth to self-medicate symptoms of depression or self-diagnosed ADHD. A probable majority of meth users take the drug to increase energy and become more productive, especially at work. Hey, what boss doesn't like increased productivity? Employees whose jobs rely on financial incentives such as commissions or bonuses face the most temptation. Others at risk include those who work on tight deadlines, such as workers in tech, advertising, law, and management.

Workers with physically demanding or highly repetitive jobs, such as professional athletes and soldiers, and tradesmen like electricians, carpenters, laborers, and drywallers, also have an incentive to use. Over the years, many of these folks have told me of casually dissolving a small amount of crystal into their morning coffee for a punch that caffeine just can't deliver. This reminds me of a cartoon in the August 22, 2005, issue of the *New Yorker* captioned "Meth doesn't upset my stomach the way coffee does."[6]

So working harder and longer can bring more cash to the increasingly strung-out employee. But having extra money in your pocket can itself be a trigger to using more new-and-improved drugs. And, human nature being what it is, associated pocket-draining activities such as barhopping, nightclubbing, frequenting commercial sex workers, and going to strip bars or "gentleman's" clubs often increase when one has more "play" money in hand.

If you are not genetically programmed for addiction, you might get by with a daily maintenance pattern of use for a long time. But it almost always comes at a price. Depression, intellectual dulling, fatigue, and sleepiness can occur with long-term use. And the chances of those sequelae occurring increases exponentially when you intensify the high by switching the route of administration from slow absorption of the drug in the gut to—take your pick—snorting, smoking, shooting, or booty bumping.

For another portion of meth users, especially in the gay community in San Francisco, it's mostly about sex. Meth is far and away the most damaging drug of abuse in the city's gay community. Unfortunately, the meth use among men with HIV infection greatly increases the rate of HIV transmission among men who have sex with men. This happens, of course, because meth lowers inhibitions and impairs in-the-moment judgment. Also, research indicates that meth may somehow accelerate the disease process in people who are already infected with HIV.

Addressing the AIDS problem in San Francisco rests on the challenge of changing sexual behavior, not unlike the situation in Africa, where HIV is mostly heterosexually transmitted. Prevention strategies must be frank about changing behaviors with respect to sex. With meth in the mix, it becomes even more difficult to convince men to have "safer" sex, which includes the use of condoms and the avoidance of sexual acts that increase the risk of HIV transmission. Meth is obviously a hell of an aphrodisiac. It increases sexual interest, self-confidence, and energy while enhancing people's sensitivity to stimuli, and it has the potential to accentuate the ecstasy of the orgasm.

Typical hooking up in the gay community is rarely done these days in bathrooms, remote areas, or bars, and is arranged most often via the Internet, where the exchange is called "party and play." In this era of webcams and downloadable videos and photos, cruising is much more likely to involve an initial cyber contact. There are dozens of party-and-play hookup sites available on the Web; one of the most popular is Manhunt. Internet cruising allows you to skip the first few steps involved in bar cruising. Boys meet physically shortly after meeting in cyberspace. The drugs come out and get consumed. Sexual interest heightens. And the games begin. If performance is an issue, which it often is (erectile dysfunction due to meth use is sometimes called "crystal dick"), then Viagra or some equivalent makes it into the mix.

The above scenario does not represent the typical gay dating scene in San Francisco. Other dating options include monogamy, open relationships, and having casual sex in which the participants do not require meth to get down to earth. But a significant minority play regularly on the party-and-play circuit. Because speed-induced horniness and sexual pleasure are so intertwined and mutually reinforcing, addiction to meth often deepens as one becomes more involved in the party-and-play scene.

In his novel *SoMa,* author Kemble Scott describes the appeal of meth when he writes how his protagonist "discovered that crystal made him able to explore sex in ways he never realized were possible. . . . In the past, sex meant working toward the climax, an expulsion of joy. On crystal, there appeared to be no destination, only a journey, one more intense than any single orgasm."[7]

Helping men learn how to have enjoyable sex without the use of crystal meth is one of the biggest challenges in their recovery from an addiction to meth. One of these men might ask, "Hot sex without crystal?" and just as quickly answer, "Yeah, right. You gotta be kidding me." However, I've talked with dozens of men over the years who have learned how to enjoy sex fully without using drugs. So it can be done. But as a psychiatrist, I can tell you most sincerely that it is very difficult to change people's behaviors.

. . .

I've not even had a chance to address the issue of sexual orientation with Mark Hill before he arrives on the doorstep of psych emergency two days later, ostensibly to get into a program. Initially he looks as if he hasn't used meth anytime recently. But the longer he sits out front in one of the Fred Flintstone chairs, the more wound up and fretful he becomes.

I soon see that my good intentions may have bred, if not a borderline disaster, then at least an existential crisis in my patient. Before long, Mr. Hill is wailing, howling, and pounding the hard rubber chair with the palm of his hand, slapping his forehead, stomping his feet, and screaming. It calls to mind African women ululating in full-on grief at yet another funeral for a young person who has died from AIDS, or the shrouded elderly women weeping and beating their chests at the Holy Land's Wailing Wall. In that moment, he is a sacred figure. Not only is he grieving over his abusive childhood, he is also grieving over humankind's fall from grace. His grieving is noticed by almost everybody in psych emergency, not a small feat considering the cacophony that rings out here both day and night. He is a big man and he is flailing.

In the old days, he might have gotten restrained. But the clinical staff on duty, even the hard-bitten ones, can see that his bereavement is proportional to an apparently gaping chasm filled with pain, shame, and fear. This is no drama play of the sort we so often see here as someone angles for attention, medication, or a bed in the hospital.

For the next twenty minutes, I sit next to Mr. Hill, offering occasional support: "It's okay, Mark, we'll get you through this, just let it go, let the pain go." As he winds down, looking like a man who's just finished running a marathon, he does not seem particularly relieved. His life has been one of demoralization and a string of disappointments, relieved only by short-lived euphoria—the result of sticking a needle loaded with methamphetamine into his vein.

I can see that this outpouring of emotion frightens him, and I'm forced to wonder if the potential benefit of getting him into a program and off meth justifies the risk of his being overwhelmed psychologically. Frankl writes, "When a man finds that it is his destiny to suffer, he will have to accept his suffering as his task; his single and unique task. No one can relieve him of his suffering or suffer in his place. His unique opportunity lies in the way in which he bears his burden."[8] But despite Frankl's opinion that a man's suffering cannot be relieved, I work under the presumption that a physician's attempt to relieve suffering is the central tenet of the practice of ethical medicine, a fundamental concept. On an emotional level, I hate to see Mr. Hill suffer like this. I know that the odds of rescuing or curing him are long, given the chronicity and severity of his illness, yet I feel a strong need to help, to alleviate his suffering.

"Hey, Mark, I do think you should stay," I say. "We have a good shot at a treatment bed tomorrow morning, and I think a live-in program offers you your best chance to get clean. If it gets to be too much, too overwhelming for you to be here, then you can ask to leave. I prefer that you stay, but I want to let you know that you're here not on a 5150 hold, but rather on a voluntary basis."

"Doc, I don't remember ever crying like that before! I don't know what hit me."

"It's hard to know for sure, Mark."

"I think I'm ready to go to sleep. Could I have a little more Seroquel?"

"You bet. I'll be back tomorrow morning, and we'll put together a plan. Get a good night's rest. It's not easy in a place like this, but just let the Scroquel do its job."

"Thanks. Sorry about that scene. I haven't cried like that since I was a kid. I'm not sure what happened there. Sorry."

"No need to apologize. I'm not sure what happened either," I say, although I am pretty sure I do know what happened. He seemed to be in the midst of a dissociative bout of grieving, marked by severe agitation, not too dissimilar from what is called a flashback within the diagnosis of post-traumatic stress disorder (PTSD). I decide to let sleeping dogs lie for now and to ask him later, if he can ever tolerate the discussion, what sense he can make of it.

Mr. Hill's outburst is not a classic type of flashback, but his intense display suggests someone who has bottled up his emotions for a long time. I am fairly certain that he has PTSD, based on his experiences as a child and a teen. And I have little doubt that he's witnessed a large amount of trauma since then. In U.S. psychiatric nosology, PTSD is classified as an anxiety disorder, on the assumption that the patient has been exposed to a severely traumatic event, outside the realm of everyday human experience, in which the "person's response involved intense fear, helplessness, or horror."[9]

Years later, the trauma can be unpredictably reexperienced via unwanted memories, nightmares, panic attacks, or flashbacks. Adding to the distress is an ongoing feeling of being on guard, unable to rest. A subtler aspect of PTSD is a person's avoidance of people, places, or things that might trigger memories of the traumatic event. And the subtlest part of PTSD is an overall numbing of responsiveness to one's environment. It seems that this is the feature of PTSD, along with associated depression, that Mark Hill is trying to inoculate himself against with his injections of methamphetamine.

Many psychiatric researchers see the dissociative aspects of PTSD as being just as important as its anxiety symptoms in understanding the disorder. Mohan Isaac and Prabhat Chand describe the phenomenon in some detail: "The common theme shared by dissociative disorders is a partial or complete loss of normal integration between memories of the past, awareness of identity, and immediate sensations and control of bodily movements. [Dissociative abilities] reflect a protective strategy that is either innate or developed in early childhood in response to anxiety-provoking or dangerous situations. Later on, such states are potentially triggered by situations that induce similar emotions of fear or anxiety."[10]

Though I had observed several bona fide dissociative episodes during my psychiatric training, mostly regressions to childlike behavior in adults who had been severely physically or sexually abused in childhood, at the time I treated Mr. Hill I'd seen only one undeniably authentic flashback. This occurred in a Vietnam combat veteran who time- and space-traveled from San Francisco circa 1991 to the hills of Vietnam circa 1968. His son had accompanied him to the emergency room of the San Francisco Veterans' Affairs Medical Center, and I was asked to evaluate him. At the time, I was a third-year psychiatric resident on call.

The man viewed the emergency room as a jungle fort and all of us, including his own son, as the enemy, as Viet Cong. Had he had a gun, he most certainly would have shot us all. Instead he cowered and cried and put his hands over his head as if he were surrendering, begging us to spare his life, to not shoot him. It was a standoff for more than fifteen minutes until he finally came out of it, remembering nothing of it.

Amnesia is a product of dissociation, which is a splitting off of the psyche performed to protect the mind, spirit, and soul from the real-time horrors befalling the body. It is a desperate defense against repetitive severe trauma. It moves both place and time from the here and now. The flashback experienced by this veteran displaced the "here" by thousands of miles, and the "now" by more than twenty years. It was a radical defense, engineered in the dimensions of space and time.

I do think Mr. Hill was in the midst of a dissociative episode in psych emergency. I hypothesize that finding himself once again in a chaotic institutional setting, albeit a relatively safe one, may have triggered memories of his traumatic childhood both at home and at the juvey camp.

. . .

The next day I'm able to get Mr. Hill a treatment bed. He lasts two days before leaving. "I was feeling cooped up."

He calls me the next Monday, while I'm seeing patients at the meth addiction outpatient clinic. I can't talk long.

"How're you doing?" I ask.

"I'm okay," he says. "I'm a survivor."

"That you are, Mark, that you are," I say.

He tells me he wants to take another stab at residential treatment. I tell him to come visit me in psych emergency at a time when he's *not* high on speed.

Two days later, he walks into the sally port of psych emergency at General Hospital. I can see instantly, through the shatterproof glass, that he's been using. He shifts from foot to foot, wiping his nose on the sleeve of his shirt. His hygiene is poor, his hair unkempt, his movements jerky. His pupils are saucer-sized. "Oh, no," I whisper to myself. "High again."

The triage nurse asks me if I know the guy. I say, sure, he's one of my patients over at the speed clinic.

"Mind talking to him, Paul?"

"Not at all."

"Hey, Mark, what's up?" I yell through the thick glass.

"I just had to see you today. I want to discuss some ideas with you."

"Are you ready to go to a residential program? Did you come here to talk about that?"

He pauses for the first time. "Well, no. It's more important than that. It's about the future of our country."

"Do you want to come in?" I ask.

"No."

"How about I come talk to you in the hallway, Mark?"

"Yeah, sure, that'd be great."

Now, if he were actually serious about getting into a residential program, then I'd damn sure bring him in, even if psych emergency was jammed to the rafters. I meet Mr. Hill in the hallway outside.

"Hi, doc, good to see you," Mr. Hill says, offering me his large hand. I shake it firmly but briefly. "Hey, can we sit outside? I'm dying for a smoke."

"Sure. Mark, I probably have only five-ten minutes, and I'll have to get back in there."

We sit down on a long wooden bench along the outside wall of the hospital under a narrow canopy. I find talking in this place of contact not so different from interviewing patients under a tree, which I occasionally did when I worked in Zimbabwe. Confidentiality might suffer if it weren't for the fact that nearly everyone gives us a wide berth.

His hair is irregularly shorn. He wears blue jeans and an untucked flannel shirt. He keeps standing up, gesturing, alternately putting on and doffing his seed-company cap over and over again. He is uncomfortably close to me, towering over me, going on and on about the world's injustices. "Where's the fuckin' outrage?" he starts, spreading spittle as he speaks. "What Bush is doing over there in Iraq? And we're just going to sleep here over it! I'm planning to march to Washington! And who's coming with me? Are you coming with me?"

I know it's the speed talking, and I know that his focus on politics conveniently keeps us from talking about his messed-up life, including his humongous drug problem. Though he is speaking loudly and fervently, I am not afraid. Here is a giant of a man, an experienced street fighter, yelling and gesticulating as he looms over me. My gut sensors of impending violence, however, are not firing. I trust him not to clock me.

It's sad that, as imposing as he looks, he is such a frightened little boy inside that six-foot-five frame. His suffering is palpable, essentially unmitigated, and he has little solace, except for, in his own mind, that provided by meth. Today, out on the bench under a hot spring sun, he is grandiose and expansive as he spouts about injustice. Each time he gets clean and sober, for no more than a week at a time, the painful reality of his past comes surging up into his consciousness. It's too terrible to be believed. The grief is too heavy. His nerves are too raw. The anger, the rage, becomes unmanageable. In these moments, when he is close to unleashing the beast, he is on the razor's edge.

"I don't really want to die, I don't really want to hurt anyone else," a shred of his conscious mind declares. "Better to take another shot, clear it out, clear it out, sweep the cobwebs, clear the deck." This is the way he so eloquently describes what meth does for him. It's unusual in that meth users more often describe the intense rush of euphoria, of lusty horniness, as the reason they shoot up. What Mr. Hill does with it is unusual and perhaps reflects a long-standing habit—he takes it not for the high but to get "well." What a strange way to deal with the psychic pain of abandonment, of abuse, of misery. He doesn't describe his habit as self-medicating his depression, as many recovering stimulant addicts do.

The meth awakens Mr. Hill, reversing the deadening, soul-destroying feelings that make up the darkest aspects of PTSD. He deeply believes that it is the methamphetamines that ease his psychic pain—"clear it out, sweep the cobwebs, clear the deck."

So that he can go on for another day.

．　．　．

I eventually lost track of Mr. Hill. He came back both to the clinic and to psych emergency a few more times, but six months later he disappeared entirely. The streets may have finally done him in, or he may have gotten snared in the jail system. In any event, I can speculate that his brief foray into psychiatric and drug treatment may have overwhelmed him. He couldn't stand to set aside his most reliable coping strategy, that of shooting speed, the one that chased his demons away, if only for a little while.

NINE

THE WITNESS

Trauma Underlies the Pain

Mary Hughlett is a twenty-two-year-old fourth-year junior at San Francisco State University. She works part-time as a café waitress in addition to taking three classes as an upper-division English major.

I see her on the day shift, the reevaluation shift. She is one of eleven patients assigned to me that morning.

"Ah, a high-functioning patient," I say to no one in particular, knowing that my interview will necessarily take anywhere from thirty minutes to an hour, which, as I've mentioned before, is an eternity in my neck of the woods. Why so long? For starters, you've got a patient who not only can talk but also is willing to talk, and, most important, who will be helped by talking, opening up, shining a light into the shadows of her psyche.

In any event, I will need to make a considered judgment concerning whether to hospitalize or release her and, furthermore, will need to justify my decision in writing. If I'm going to discharge her, I will need to construct a strong rationale with a solid outpatient treatment plan. Conversely, if I hospitalize her—someone who is young, new to the system, and essentially "normal" at her baseline—I must be certain that this will be more a help than a harm to her in the long run.

I breeze through her chart, looking specifically at the strength of the 5150 hold, written by a member of the SFPD, and the impression and plan noted by my overnight colleague. A paper trail littered with a damning 5150, suggesting a highly lethal patient, makes discharge more difficult. In contrast, a vaguely written document, a "weak 5150," more easily paves the way for discharge. Police officers, who are not psychiatrically trained beyond a basic four-hour "5150 orientation," often prepare 5150s of the latter variety. Furthermore, if the overnight doctor documents the patient as a high risk with a definite need for inpatient psychiatric admission, then my hands are essentially tied. In that situation, I must have my ducks in a row to justify a patient's release.

In Ms. Hughlett's case, despite a graphic description of blood on the premises, the SFPD officer did not comment on her intention in cutting herself: "Upon arrival to the subject's apartment, I noticed blood on the bathroom floor and razors scattered about. The subject had a blood-soaked towel on her wrist. The subject was crying and screaming. She said, 'I can't take it anymore. I just want it over with.'"

Though this is a lucid description of the situation, it is not one that screams out "needs to be hospitalized for weeks." I guess he felt that the blood would do the talking. Furthermore, the night-shift doctor summarized her note with the standard "overnight and reeval" recommendation, telegraphing that she didn't see the patient's acute suicide risk as being anything more than moderate, for which discharge with a strong outpatient plan might be more than adequate. There are many days in which I'd rather do the quick ten-minute interview and conclude, "Yes, you're good to go" or "Sorry, miss, but I'm sending you upstairs to a watered-down version of *Cuckoo's Nest.*"

I guess it's no surprise that I was a center in football and a catcher in baseball: I always want to work in the middle, to get my hands on the ball, to see the complexity, to get my psyche revved and my hands dirty, to wallow in the confusion that is human existence. And, in front of me, Ms. Mary Hughlett provides me with an opportunity to do some good. I know it sounds terrible to say that seeing someone who's just sliced open a prominent vein of the wrist, earning her some deep suturing and a monumental pressure bandage, is a routine thing, but for me I'm afraid it's become so.

I see the entire spectrum of patients in psych emergency. Though a writer friend of mine described my work as a parade of "dumpster-diving, Thunderbird-swilling winos" and other such characters, fairly often I evaluate educated upper-middle-class people who are, by most estimations, having the worst day of their lives. Many of these patients are college students. I've seen students from all the educational institutions in the Bay Area—City College, SF State, UC Berkeley, Stanford, Hastings College of Law, and USF, as well as UCSF students from the nursing, pharmacy, dentistry, and medicine departments.

And what might prompt an educated middle- to upper-middle-class young woman to deeply slice her wrist? Usually it's a combo deal. It's often about things like out-of-control alcohol use, academic stress, family pressures, untreated depression, trauma issues, and rocky "coming out" issues. But it almost always includes major relationship issues—infidelity, breakups, arguments, domestic violence.

. . .

I sit down with Ms. Hughlett in the interview room. She looks
her stated age. She is dressed in a blood-spattered hospital gown.
A lumpy soft gauze wrap covers her left wrist and forearm. Her
dark brown eyes migrate often toward the floor as we talk. "The
main question, I guess, is 'Why now?'" I start. "What's been
happening in your life that may have contributed to you hurting
yourself like this?"

"Well." She pauses. "That's a good question. I just broke up
with my boyfriend. He wouldn't stop smoking weed, and I had
asked him to not smoke when he was with me. But he liked to
get high before we had sex. Our sex life was pretty strong. But I
had to wonder if I wasn't exciting enough for him without
drugs. Why did he need a drug for us to be sexual?"

"How long had you guys been dating?"

"About six months. I think he was seeing other girls. I can't
prove it. Of course, he denies it. I feel pretty good about my
decision. I mean, I was the one who broke up with him. I
thought I would be okay. But last night I guess I got to feeling
really lonely. I felt really, really nervous, and then something
happened. I kind of snapped, now that I think about it. I started
crying hysterically, and then the details get all fuzzy—until I
woke up in the emergency room with some intern sewing up
my wrist."

"So how did you leave it with your boyfriend—do you still
talk to him?"

"No, he's really pissed at me. I think he's been talking shit
about me. Well, I say, 'Fuck him.' I don't need him."

This could be false bravado, uttered by someone who is
absolutely terrified of being left behind. But I don't think so.

Ms. Hughlett's attitude is so different from that of a person with borderline personality disorder after the breakup of a relationship. First and foremost, a person with borderline personality disorder is usually the one who gets dumped—one who is likely to hang on even when the handwriting is on the wall. The hallmark of a borderline personality is a fear of real or imagined abandonment.

Unfortunately, we see many patients who suffer from full-blown borderline personality disorder in psych emergency. According to psychiatrist John Rouse, an expert on personality disorders in emergency psychiatry, "Borderlines and emergency services represent a 'good fit' since both are by their very nature action oriented."[1] These patients suffer from an unstable sense of self, low self-esteem, tempestuous relationships, problems with impulse control, and anger issues. They either idealize or devalue others, feel depressed or preoccupied with death, and cut or burn themselves for psychological reasons. They engender strong feelings in others, including psychiatrists-in-training. They make others want to punish them or rescue them. Even experienced therapists fall prey to the insults and charms of the borderline personality.

We see a few of these patients on a regular basis in psych emergency. They are among those who compulsively go to the Golden Gate Bridge and ponder jumping. Or who repeatedly cut their wrists or burn themselves. Or who bang their heads and scratch themselves in psych emergency, necessitating the use of seclusion and restraints to maintain safety.

For patients with severe borderline personality disorder, psych emergency provides a container for acting out. "There are four key elements of the PES 'holding environment': nurture, limits, consistency, and communication," writes Rouse.[2]

Ms. Hughlett impresses me as a genuinely tough person. It's impossible to say for sure at the moment, but my gut tells me that her resilience in the face of abandonment was not an act. I'm sure she has her soft spots, her weaknesses—we all do—but she also demonstrates a kind of hardiness, buoyancy even, for someone who, I am speculating, has had a hard life. "So how is your wrist feeling?" I ask.

"It doesn't really hurt," she says. Her voice is soft, sweet, slow.

"Did they give you any pain meds?"

"Yeah, some ibuprofen. It helped a little." She pauses. I wait, slowing my breath, averting my gaze, resonating with her in the moment. I do this automatically when I sit and talk with patients, a habit practiced over many years.

"But it's the emotional pain I can't take anymore." She again hesitates. She studies her feet in their hospital-issued polyester-knit brown booties.

"What kind of emotional pain?" I ask.

Her eyes mist. "I'm sorry," she whispers.

I wait. "It's okay to cry," I say.

"Well, in my family it wasn't," she says, her voice rising, her features animating. "I would get punished for crying—even if I got stung by a bee or skinned my knee. I think my mother was embarrassed. She always worried a lot about what other people would think of us."

While she talks, I look more closely at Ms. Hughlett's physical presence and features. She is short, about five foot one, with brown skin. I can't ascertain her racial background. Of course, this isn't of primary importance, but a consideration of culture and ethnicity is part of a comprehensive evaluation.

"Where'd you grow up?"

"L.A. Out in the Valley, actually."

"Who was in your family?"

"Well, my mom and dad split when I was two. I didn't see much of him until my teenage years. So I was raised, if you want to call it that, by my mom and my stepdad."

"Any siblings?"

"Yeah, two half brothers. They're younger. One's in fifth grade and the other eighth."

"Oh, little brothers," I say. "I bet they're annoying."

Ms. Hughlett allows herself a half smile. "Oh, yeah, especially when they were rug rats. Now that they're a little older, they're too cool to even talk to me."

"So how do you get along with your mother nowadays?"

"Well, we don't talk much. She's mad at me for coming up here to go to school. It's just that I needed to get away. To put it bluntly, doctor, my mom is an enabler. My stepfather used to be a nasty drunk. Like, when I was in middle school, she either couldn't or wouldn't protect me from him."

"Protect you?" I ask. "Protect you from what?"

"He was verbally abusive when he got drunk, which was pretty much every day. My mom was working. He wasn't. He'd just sit at home and drink beer all day. He'd be messed up by the time I got home from school. He'd call me racial names, tell me I was a slut, tell me I'd never amount to anything, tell me I was stupid. This was even though I got all As and Bs throughout school. I was a good student!" Her voice rises, her lips curl at the thought.

"See, he never loved me. I think in part because I didn't look like him. I was my father's daughter. I wasn't white." She sneers. "He used to call me half-breed. See, my mom came here from the Philippines when she was nine. And she is half-Filipina, half-white. My grandfather was a GI from North Dakota, of all places, and my grandma lived in a village. My father was half African American, half Native American, from Oklahoma. Unfortunately, he ruined his life with alcohol and drugs. He died last year; his liver gave out. He was only forty-three.

"So, doctor, as you can see, I'm no half-breed. Hell no, I'm a quarter-breed!" she says, laughing. She is beginning to mobilize her affect, her emotional connectivity. "A quarter Filipina, a quarter white, a quarter black, and a quarter Native American— Choctaw, I think.

"And my stepdad, as you can imagine, is white, no offense. I don't know what happened to him. The bottle, I guess. I mean, he grew up in a liberal family. He's a smart guy. He has a master's degree. He's had some very good jobs over the years. But after my mom got pregnant with Oscar, he kind of lost it. My mom can't lay down the law. She works two jobs to keep the household going. And my brothers? They're video game zombies. They come home from school, grab a snack, and then hit their Xboxes for hours on end. My stepfather doesn't give a shit."

This kind of openness and insightfulness is one of the things that, over the years, has kept me coming back to work in the psych ER. It is my privilege to hear her story. I need to hear her story. The more I know about her, the better my decision— about what to do, how to help her—will be. My time with her is an oasis from the madness. I can put on my trusty psychodynamo hat and pretend I am in an office in San Francisco's so-called shrink row on Sacramento or Union Street. I can put my private hospital experience to work. Mary Hughlett is no dumpster-diving wino, no sirree.

The textbook scenario for performing a crisis assessment would by now have me cutting the patient off to ask linear, telegraphic questions such as "When you cut your wrist, were you intending to die?" and then get to the psychosocial history later in the interview, if at all. But one of the finest bits of supervisory advice I've gotten over the years? "Follow the patient's lead. Go where she goes and you'll learn so much in so little time." Now, of course, this advice can take you on a bridge to nowhere if you've got a patient who is rambling or going off on tangents or mumbling only monosyllabic answers. But following the lead of a patient like Ms. Hughlett is like mining for gold.

"You know, Mary, I'm impressed with how well you seem to know yourself, at such a young age. What do you make of that?"

I can almost see her blush. "Well, it's not because I've had any therapy, that's for sure. Though I'm sure I could use some." She glances at me sheepishly, laughing before looking downward. It seems as if she is asking me to assure her she doesn't need therapy. This I cannot do.

"I think it's because I'm a survivor," she adds. "I've had to put up with a lot of shit. Go through a lot of things on my own." Her face turns almost ashen. She hangs her head. Her speech slows. She shuts down.

I pause. My voice lowers. "What kind of things?"

"Well, my dad's death hit me pretty hard. We weren't all that close, but we looked alike—my skin is pretty dark, my eyes are like his. Probably why my stepfather hated me so much. And my dad, my dad was really well read. He dropped out of high school and got his GED, but he read everything he could get his hands on—from *Scientific American* to the *Economist* to Dickens and political books of the day. I'm a voracious reader, too," she says.

I pause to gather my thoughts. It's getting to a sort of crunch time. I shift gears in the interview so we can get to the nitty-gritty of the suicide risk assessment. Eventually I will return to an exploration of her psychological mindedness—to assess her willingness and readiness to embark on a course of psychotherapy with, ideally, a caring, capable therapist not long after she leaves psych emergency.

Between my chart review and a series of closed-end questions, I am able to obtain some semblance of a risk assessment. Among the variables associated with an increased risk, it is probable that she suffers from what we call a major mood- or anxiety-related illness. She likely suffers from major depression with some overlay of anxiety, perhaps even a full-blown post-traumatic stress disorder. And it is a pretty serious cut—she nearly required a tendon repair. If her symptoms of anxiety, depression, and proneness to dissociation continue to go untreated, she is more likely to again do something self-injurious on impulse. This behavior could lead to even greater hazard, even lethality.

On the mitigating side, the slashing was done impulsively, without premeditation. She doesn't drink alcohol or use drugs. The lack of substance abuse in the picture greatly reduces her risk. She called 911 herself after she woke up from what can effectively be called a trance state. She denies suicidal ideation, intent, or a plan for it now. While she has episodically and passively wished to be dead, she denies any prior history of suicide attempts. She's never been admitted to a psych ward before. She is not psychotic.

In a consideration of her suicide risk, the fact that she sliced herself while in the midst of a dissociative state cuts both ways, no pun intended. The positive side is that she did not consciously plan this suicide attempt far in advance. The negative aspect is that, if she dissociates once again during a stressful time in her life, she may do something dangerous again. But obviously I cannot justify holding her against her will just to prevent her from dissociating again.

Her acute risk of suicide falls in the low to moderate range. I will need a solid discharge plan in order to justify releasing her from psych emergency. I will also need to screen her for a history of physical or sexual abuse. Red flags for a history of abuse or neglect have already been raised, including her current self-injury, a verbally abusive, alcoholic stepfather, and an easily shamed, enabling mother. These issues matter because their presence in the psychiatric history is such a high predictor of post-traumatic stress disorder and borderline personality disorder. Identifying either of these psychiatric problems would substantially inform the construction of a long-term treatment plan from which she could benefit. I don't get the sense that she has a borderline personality disorder, but I do think she may have PTSD, for which I will screen her. The probable lack of a personality disorder really improves her prognosis.

For all the personal questions that we as psychiatrists are called on to ask, screening for childhood abuse entails asking some of the thorniest ones, but also some of the most important. I start: "The next question might be a little harder for you to talk about. But I wouldn't ask you if it wasn't important to your getting through this. It's entirely up to you if you want to answer it."

"Okay."

"Did your stepfather ever beat you physically?"

She pauses. "No. He threatened me with violence a few times, but he never really hit me."

"Did he ever touch you in ways you didn't like?"

Ms. Hughlett freezes. I wait. Within seconds, she breaks down sobbing.

"I'm sorry this is so hard for you," I say quietly. I wait some more.

This is the question that overwhelms the proverbial dam of her defenses. I try to err on the side of not prying unnecessarily, but this issue may very well be the eight-hundred-pound gorilla in this young woman's life. It might be a contributing factor to the current crisis—a 911 call, a bloody bathroom, a trip to the county ER, deep sutures, a trip in soft restraints to psych emergency, an awakening next to commercial sex workers, intravenous drug users, registered sex offenders, and street-hardened folks, with the chronically psychotic thrown in for good measure.

Odds are that this is Mary Hughlett's first and last visit to a place like this. And, frankly, if I think that closely questioning her can do anything to minimize her chances of bouncing back to a place like this, how can I do otherwise? Chances are excellent that I will never see her again, so I can't ignore this issue now. If I address it with her, she will have a chance to deal with it in the future. So it behooves me to use my forty-five minutes with her in a wise fashion. My goal is to give her an introduction to the world of mental health that does not perpetuate her trauma, that helps her turn her life even a few degrees left or right, to get her on a path to what I call having a regular life. This includes the pursuit of life, love, liberty, work, and even happiness.

She collects herself, looking down all the while, wiping her tears away with the back of her unbandaged hand. I offer her a tissue.

"Yes, the bastard. For a year and a half, the first time before I ran away from home, he used to force himself on me every day. It started with him just threatening me and me having to give him a hand job. Then he stuck his penis in my mouth. My God, I was only ten. I didn't know what to do. It was so sick. He would say, 'Just suck on it like a lollipop. Doesn't it taste good?' He would start to moan and then . . ."

She looks away. Her facial expression is bland. "That is so awful," I say. "You poor girl. No one should have to experience something like that."

Ms. Hughlett is remarkably calm and focused as she continues: "Finally when I was eleven—I was in the sixth grade, I think—I stopped coming home after school, skipping dinner and then staying out late. I spent a lot of nights at my friend's house. Her parents were great. They didn't know exactly what was happening, but I think they knew it was something bad. My mother was pissed. She said I was an evil girl."

"Did you ever tell your mother about the sexual abuse?"

"Well, I tried to, but she would end up yelling at me and calling me disrespectful. She would say, 'You crazy girl, don't go around making up lies about my husband.'"

"Talk about getting shut down," I say. "Learning you couldn't trust the very person who was supposed to be taking care of you and looking out for your best interests."

"Well, I don't want to make excuses for her, but this was during a very hard time for her. I'm sure she was depressed. I know she was way moody most of her life. My brothers were little and she was working a lot. My stepfather finally got off his fat ass and got some low-level assistant manager job that at least got us benefits."

"How else did you deal with this situation?"

"Well, I was lucky. My friend would listen to me. We could cry together if I needed that."

"Yes, that kind of support is important," I say. "Did your stepfather hurt you after that?"

"A few times, yeah. He cornered me, even though I avoided him like the plague. He would say, 'Let me have you again. You're dirty. You're ruined for life. Your mother said you told her that I was molesting you. Ha! She didn't believe you. She thinks you're bad, too.'

"'Fuck you!' I said at the time, and I punched him," she says, smiling at the memory. "Drew blood, too. He never touched me again after that. He never told my mom that I smacked him a good one either. I think I scared him a little bit. I hope so. The coward."

. . .

Researchers estimate that up to 30 percent of women have experienced some form of sexual abuse during their lifetimes.[3] Among this group of women, approximately seven out of ten develop a psychiatric disorder in adulthood—specifically major depression, panic disorder, post-traumatic stress disorder, borderline personality disorder, an eating disorder, or substance abuse—when compared to women who have not been abused.[4] What differentiates the women who are afflicted with psychiatric problems as adults from those who are spared has been a matter of great interest to social science researchers.

According to some researchers, "More than just the 'flip side' of a risk factor, the notion of resilience encompasses psychological and biological characteristics, intrinsic to an individual, that might be modifiable and that confer protection against the development of psychopathology in the face of stress."[5] Another way of conceptualizing resilience is through the term "hardiness," which has been defined as "a stable personality resource that consists of three psychological attitudes and cognitions: commitment, challenge, and control. . . . 'Commitment' refers to an ability to turn events into something meaningful and important. 'Control' refers to the belief that, with effort, individuals can influence the course of events around them. 'Challenge' refers to a belief that fulfillment in life results from the growth and wisdom gained from difficult or challenging experiences."[6]

The biological aspect of resilience suggests that some people's brains are temperamentally wired to more easily absorb stress, tolerate anxiety, resist mood dampening, and dissociate easily while reintegrating seamlessly. As one can imagine, accessing these biological attributes in a time of need is much easier said than done.

. . .

"We've covered some pretty difficult terrain here, Mary. How are you doing with all of this—how are you feeling right now?" I ask.

"Well, I'm a little freaked out. I'm still sad, a little bit nervous. But I do feel better. I haven't talked to anyone else about this—except for two of my oldest, dearest girlfriends, no one else knows about it."

"Those are some intense experiences to keep bottled up inside. It can be unpredictable how those kinds of things will bubble up on a person."

"Now that you mention it, I did feel an almost out-of-body experience right before I cut myself. I just felt totally weird, like I wasn't myself, like it was somebody else cutting my arm, not really me."

"I'd have to say that your alter ego really did a number on your forearm—you nicked your tendon but thankfully missed the artery and nerve nearby. Lucky for you, you didn't end up in emergency surgery."

"Yeah, you're right."

"What you experienced sounds very much like something called dissociation—literally disconnecting your mind from your body. It can happen when people drink too much alcohol, what's referred to as a 'blackout.'"

"I don't drink," she quickly adds. "Knowing my dad's history, seeing how crazy it makes my stepfather."

"Dissociation also occurs in people who've been traumatized. And what you went through would certainly qualify. Dissociation is a way of splitting your mind away from your body—it's a way of escaping an intolerable situation in the moment."

Ms. Hughlett starts crying again.

"What are you experiencing?" I ask.

"It's just that . . . that now I remember doing that when I was ten. I would put myself up in the corner of the room and watch, like a disinterested observer, what was happening just down below."

"My goodness, what else could you have done? It's just such a breach of trust, for an adult, a parent, for chrissakes, to take advantage of you like that. How does it make you feel to think about it right now?"

"Really pissed," she says, "and really sad, too. So I'm pretty messed up, huh, doc?"

"I wouldn't put it that way. You've done remarkably well in your life considering the burden you've carried all these years— mostly alone. You've shown a lot of courage, in fact."

"You think so?" she asks.

"Absolutely. Moving up here as a teenager on your own. Finding your own place, working to support yourself, paying your rent, paying your tuition. Not falling back on alcohol and drugs, when many others in your situation have."

Though I haven't told her yet, I am beginning to feel comfortable with the notion of discharging her if she agrees to follow up with a therapist within a few days of leaving the emergency room.

She breaks into a small smile. "Yeah, I guess you're right. I don't usually think of myself as having accomplished anything. Thank you."

"You're welcome, Mary," I say. "You've suffered a lot. You're only twenty-two. I hope you have a long life ahead of you—a career, a relationship, a family, if you want that."

"Yes, yes, I do. I do want all of those things," she says, "at some point."

"That's good. You're bright, you're young, you're gutsy. You have a lot of potential." She seems a good candidate for psychotherapy—intelligent, open, insightful (especially for someone so young). But is she motivated? Would this wrist cut, a new experience for her, be enough motivation to get her involved in psychotherapy? Or are her issues buried too deeply—too submerged by her mostly adaptive defense mechanisms? These are questions in search of answers.

"All the staff's been really nice here, but some of the other people here have gotten me weirded out. Sorry."

"Hey, I don't blame you," I say. "This is a pretty intense environment. And many of these people are pretty sick."

"What do you say? Can I go home? I need to clean up. Put some real clothes on."

"If I were in your shoes, I'd want to get the hell out of here, too. That's normal. That's a good sign. I think I'm going to be able to let you go. . . . "

"You mean today?" she interrupts, her face lighting up.

"Yeah, probably in the next hour or so. But I want to talk to you about what's next for you on the outside. What are your plans for tomorrow, for the next week?"

"Well, I have to clean up my apartment. And I think I'll need to drop two of my three classes and get to studying and writing a paper for my third."

"Are you up to it?"

"Yeah. In a funny kind of way, I'm now more ready than ever just to get back to my plain old boring life again. To focus on school again. To steer clear of guys for a while. Work on myself a little bit."

"How do you feel about seeing a therapist sooner rather than later? I do think you have depression with some anxiety thrown in for good measure."

She hesitates. "Well . . ."

"I know therapy can seem kind of strange, and definitely intense. But I think, if nothing else, it will give you a forum, an outlet for all those frightening things bottled up inside of you."

"That's what I've been trying to avoid, though."

"Yeah, and it seemed to rear its ugly head in a most unpleasant way. You're stuck in a place like this with a deep gash in your arm, lots of blood loss. I don't mean to be too harsh, but I think that the sexual abuse at the hands of your stepfather and the emotional abuse by your mother had a fair amount to do with your cutting and your arrival here. It provided a background, and your breakup pushed you over the top."

"Yeah, doctor, I think you're right."

"A good therapist will not push you any faster than you're ready to go. You can start with your student health service, and I can give you some referrals as well. You also will need to come back to the Wound Clinic upstairs in a week or so to get those sutures removed. I'll get you an appointment."

Her face brightens. "And then I can go?"

"Yup," I say as I get out of my chair, extending my hand to shake hers. "I will bless you for takeoff." I wave an unofficial sign of the cross in the air in front of me—just like my priest used to do. "I'll inform your nurse that I've deemed you 'good to go,' and she will come and check you out of here. Should be no more than ten or fifteen minutes."

"Thank you, doctor."

"You're welcome," I say.

"This wasn't as bad as I thought."

"No?"

And, I think, that's about as good as it gets in psych emergency.

TEN

THE JUDGE

Playing God from a Psychiatric Standpoint

I'm working on the psychiatric consult service when I get a stat
page. "This is Dr. Sokol," the voice says. It belongs to none other
than the division chief of hepatology and medical director of the
liver transplant service at a private hospital where I worked for
two years.

I return the call as soon as I can. "Hi, Bob, this is Paul. You
rang? I wasn't expecting to hear straight from the boss."

"Well, it's my day on service. We really need your help on
this one."

"What's up?"

"The patient's name is Melissa Peters. She's a twenty-four-
year-old woman with no prior history of liver disease, a history
of depression, alcohol abuse, and personality disorder, who was
transferred to us from Modesto General Hospital after she took
an overdose of Tylenol. Estimated to be about thirty thousand
grams; her first blood level was 275, and her AST and ALT have
been rising, up into the 6,000s. She's in the unit, precautionary.
It's still too early to tell if she'll need a transplant. She's kind of

near the threshold. She's getting aggressive Mucomyst treatment. We'll need your advice about her suicide risk and what kind of a candidate she might be for a liver transplant." The patient's liver is failing, based on the rapidly rising tests of liver function—her AST and ALT. Mucomyst is the product name for acetylcysteine, a medicine that works as an antidote to lessen or prevent injury of the liver due to acetaminophen ingestion.

"Does she have family with her?"

"Yes, her mother. She's a good historian, a nervous wreck, of course, but a good source. Her boyfriend is here, also. He seems a bit dubious."

"Do we know anything about the circumstances of the overdose?"

"Yeah, there's a psych note from Modesto, a lot of detail in there, and I think the phone number of her therapist. She's on a 5150, due to expire day after tomorrow, and we have a sitter with her. Medical ICU—bed 22."

"All right, Bob. I'll be up before noon."

"I appreciate your help, Paul. Talk to you later."

Though I have become accustomed to evaluating physically ill patients on the medical-surgical wards of the hospital, I still find my visits to the intensive care unit disconcerting. Maybe it's the proximity to the precipice of death. Maybe it is the dispassionate way that physicians and nurses comport themselves in that setting. They're not exactly hardened, uncompassionate, or uncaring, but they're efficient and, out of necessity, take death at face value.

I slink onto the unit, the only doctor not wearing a white coat. I wear a somewhat ill-fitting navy blue blazer with khaki pants, a white oxford shirt, and a brightly colored hand-painted tie that my wife purchased for me in Africa.

I sit down at the nursing station, essentially invisible to the attendings, residents, interns, nurses, respiratory therapists, and other personnel buzzing about the place, and pick up Melissa Peters's chart and begin reading. I flip to the psych note, which, mercifully, has been dictated and typed instead of scrawled illegibly. It's pretty thorough. As I read, I feel a lump rising in my gut. The psychiatrist in Modesto has identified a number of red flags. These data points include the patient's previous episodes of self-injury and suicide attempts; her recent history of binge drinking; the fact that she's unemployed and living with her boyfriend, who seems to be verbally abusive, at a minimum; and her history of erratic behavior and, at one point, of being incarcerated for solicitation.

I enter the room. Melissa Peters is awake but drowsy, only a few lines and tubes obscuring a pretty face and bright red hair that's pulled back. She is very pale, with a subtle yellow tinge. A middle-aged woman only a bit older than me sits in a chair in the corner, working on a book of crossword puzzles. A bearded young man dressed in a flannel shirt and jeans stands near the woman, his arms crossed, his face expressionless.

"Hi," I try to say to all three of them, making eye contact with each sequentially. "My name is Dr. Linde. I'm the psychiatrist who works with the liver transplant team. Dr. Sokol and the surgeons asked me to evaluate the situation." Not my smoothest introduction, but it will have to do.

"Well, I'm her boyfriend, doctor, name's Scott, and I don't quite see why a psychiatrist is needed here. She's not crazy!" He sneers slightly while his voice stays even.

"A pleasure meeting you, Scott," I say. I offer my right hand. Scott shakes it with a near-crushing grasp. "No one is suggesting that she is," I say. "It's routine. Plus, since she overdosed, I need to assess her risk of suicide."

The middle-aged woman rises. She is moderately overweight and has a kind, round face. "Thank you for your help, doctor. My name's Doreen—I'm Missy's mother." She is dressed in black polyester slacks and a bright floral top. Her hair is done up in tight-ringed curls; dark circles surround her eyes. Her benignity provides a sharp counterpoint to Scott.

"Nice to meet you, ma'am," I say, shaking her hand.

"And you must be Ms. Peters," I say to the young woman in the bed, turning my head to look her in the eye.

"Yes, I am. I'm afraid I caused this whole mess." She lies still, seeming to concentrate on the matter at hand.

"How are you feeling physically?" I start.

"Tired, just really, really tired. And my stomach hurts like crazy."

"What have the liver doctors told you about your situation?"

"Well, they say my liver numbers are runnin' awful high and they're not sure what's gonna happen. They're hoping the liver will recover on its own. . . ."

Her voice trails off. I wait a bit before asking, "And what do they say if your liver doesn't recover on its own?"

"That I might need a transplant."

"That's true. I'm here partially because MediCal requires that all transplant candidates undergo a psychiatric evaluation before getting a liver assigned. But I'm also here because we want to figure out what happened and try to make sure that you're safe when you go home."

. . .

Deciding whether a patient is an "appropriate" candidate to receive a liver transplant is the closest that a psychiatrist gets to playing God as a doctor. Surgeons do not like to transplant livers into people with a high risk of self-destructing. This represents just another bad outcome, just another way that a transplanted liver can fail, as far as the team and the transplant surgeon are concerned. When assessing a potential organ recipient, a transplant team must formally address several practical questions:

Does the candidate have a sufficient network of family members or others to offer him or her support?

If the candidate is a recovering alcoholic or addict, what is the risk that he or she will relapse?

How compliant will the patient be?

What other medical or psychiatric problems might compromise the long-term outcome of the transplant?

How well do the patient and his or her support network understand the process?

Will the patient and his or her support network be able to work cooperatively with the team as a whole?

These issues need to be considered because of a relative scarcity of livers available for transplant nationwide. Larger questions, which operate in a complex ethical arena, include these:

How do scarce resources get allocated?

Who is entitled to them?

Who does not make the cut?

How do you place a value on an individual's life?

How do you balance the rights and needs of the individual patient, the donor and his or her family, and patients who remain on a long waiting list?

The demand for donated livers is much greater than the supply. It is estimated that nearly fifteen thousand livers are needed for transplant on an annual basis, but according to the United Network of Organ Sharing, the liver donation rate is only fifty-nine per one million people. The organization has calculated that the "death rate among those awaiting liver transplantation is 23%."[1]

Bioethicists have examined these issues in some detail. In their book, *The Ethics of Organ Transplants,* Arthur Caplan and Daniel Coelho write, "Our desire to rescue the sick conflicts with our desire to do the greatest good for the greatest number of persons with scarce resources. . . . Two prevailing principles of organ distribution divide the transplant community."[2] The first is that one must maximize efficiency, utilizing organs preferentially for those with the best chance for a good outcome. The second principle is that one must consider the urgency of need—that is, give preference to patients who are critically ill and in imminent danger of death without a transplant. Most transplant programs base their decisions on urgency of need, but these priorities are often in flux at both the local and national levels. The decisions are necessary because "liver transplantation uses a nonrenewable, absolutely scarce resource—a donor liver."[3]

Certain body organs are more readily available because they can be donated by living persons. These include kidneys, parts of pancreases, and bone marrow. Organs that cannot be harvested until the donor has died are in much shorter supply. These include livers, hearts, lungs, and retinas.

Kidneys are most readily available. Since humans have two kidneys, and one can be spared, well-matched living donors can often be found. Moreover, dialysis allows many transplant candidates to live for extended periods while awaiting a donor. The postsurgical results are usually excellent for both donor and recipient, with an expected one-year success rate of about 90 percent among recipients.

Hearts are much scarcer because the organ is more likely to be irretrievably damaged in the process of the donor's passing. And unlike with lung transplants, in which one lobe can be donated, or pancreatic transplants, in which a piece of the organ can be transplanted, a heart transplant works only when the entire organ remains intact, with viable tissue.

The vast majority of patients who require liver transplant for survival suffer from cirrhosis, which occurs when soft, healthy, functional liver tissue is progressively replaced by hard, nodular, dysfunctional tissue. As this occurs, its ability to detoxify and metabolize progressively deteriorates. Chronic severe alcohol abuse and infection with the hepatitis C virus are the most common causes of end-stage cirrhosis. Once a person stops drinking, the liver has a remarkable capacity for recovery, but only up to a point.

In the case of hepatitis C, if the virus does not respond to aggressive antiviral treatment, generally interferon and ribavirin, then over time the liver may develop fibrosis, and this may progress to cirrhosis. And that's when patients develop nausea, bloating, confusion, and jaundice, hallmarks of end-stage liver disease. Deficiencies in clotting can lead to bleeding problems.

Kidney failure can be a late complication. Many hepatitis C patients become infected with the virus as a result of sharing needles with other injection-drug users. And many injection-drug users are also heavy drinkers, making for a double whammy of cirrhosis caused by the combination of alcoholic liver disease and hepatitis C infection.

Most patients with cirrhosis are sick for an extended time before they actually require a liver transplant to survive. Because of this, the liver transplant team has a long time to get to know a candidate. But when it comes to the fulminants—those with severe, acute liver failure—the team does not have this luxury. The decision-making process undertaken to answer the question "Is this person an appropriate candidate for transplant or not?" gets compressed.

Among the dramatic causes of liver failure are ingestion of the death cap mushroom, *Amanita phalloides,* and overdosing on acetaminophen, the chemical name for Tylenol, the over-the-counter pain reliever that is universally taken. According to one researcher, "About 200 persons a year die of fulminant hepatic failure from acetaminophen overdosage. Approximately half of the overdoses are intentional."[4] So the big question for the "liver psychiatrist" in these situations is: "Will this person attempt or 'succeed' at suicide in the future?"

. . .

"Have you ever been admitted to a psychiatric ward?"

"Well, twice. The first was when I was a teenager and I was cutting myself and putting out cigarettes on my arms."

"And how was it being in the hospital?"

"Oh, that time, pretty cool. I stayed for about three weeks. I made a few friends, but by the time I left they had all abandoned me. And a lot of cute guys—this was before Scott, of course."

"And what about the second time?"

Her face grows dim. "It was at Modesto General—what a snake pit. I was only in there for about three days before they kicked me out of there. I never got the help I needed."

"What do you mean?"

"Well, they kept telling me how I needed to stop drinkin' or else it was gonna kill me. They wanted to send me to an alcohol program. I refused. Plus, the doctor said he wouldn't refill my Xanax prescription—he said I was an addict and shouldn't be on tranquilizers."

"How'd you end up in the hospital that time?"

"Well, that was what, Mom, a year and a half ago?"

"Yeah, about that—early last year."

"I had just broken up with a guy who was such an asshole. He used to throw me up against the wall, push me around. He even socked me in the jaw once. But Scott took care of him, didn't you, honey?"

"Yeah, babe, it was worth going to jail for forty-five days to get even with that guy."

Mama Peters looks at the floor, sighing and shaking her head.

"Well, I was cryin' all the time, drinkin' more than usual. The Prozac wasn't workin'. So I just got fed up and cut myself."

"Where?"

She pulls her hands out from underneath the covers and flings her wrists above her in a rapid, smooth motion. "See, doc. Look at all of 'em. But that big one there—on that one I was tryin' to kill myself. I used a razor blade, tried to slice into my artery. Only hit my vein, though. I still made a helluva mess."

I examine the flexor side of her left forearm—the part most accessible to a weapon procured in the right hand. An angry-looking scar extends from the palm of her hand to the middle of her forearm.

"Yup, that one," she says, almost proudly. "I cut the tendon, just missed the nerve, lost about three pints of blood, had to go to surgery to fix it up."

"How about all those other cuts?" I ask, referring to the dozens of half-inch to two-inch horizontal scars. "Were you trying to kill yourself with those cuts?"

"Naw, I just needed to release the pain, get some help somewhere. I know it sounds crazy, but I feel calmer after I cut myself."

"No, Ms. Peters, not crazy at all. I've talked to a lot of other people who injure themselves for the same reason. Your body releases natural painkillers—substances called endorphins, and they seem to promote a sense of well being. So, have you taken another overdose, jumped off something, taken a gun to yourself, tried hanging yourself?" I know it sounds like a grisly laundry list, and it is, but a psychiatrist sometimes has to spell out a list of methods to jog people's memories.

"Oh, no, nothing like any of those."

"Do you own a gun?"

Ms. Peters squirms a bit in her bed. She stammers, "Uh . . . I . . . I . . . I don't have a gun."

"Is there one in your household?"

Scott jumps in then. "Yeah, doc, I own a shotgun, a .16 gauge, use it for duck huntin'. Any law against that?"

"No. But having a gun in a household raises the risk of an accidental death by about fortyfold."

"The gun is locked in a cabinet," says Scott. "It's not loaded. The ammo is locked up in a different place."

"Good," I say. "Sounds like you've taken all the important safety precautions. So, Melissa, what was going on before this overdose?"

"We've been under a lot of stress. I'm not working—I got fired from my part-time job as a cashier because I got into too many arguments with the customers and also with the manager. I'm lookin' for another one, but I don't want to stoop to tele-marketing. And Scott, well he's a freelance mechanic and he's kinda between jobs, so money is really, really tight. We're already a month behind on the rent. We'd have nowhere to go if we got kicked out. My mom would let me stay with her, but she won't let me and Scott live together under her roof."

"Hey, it's her place, it's her decision," he says, shooting a malign glance at Doreen Peters. "We're adults. We should be able to take care of ourselves." He nearly growls as he says this.

"And me and Scott, we're engaged. We have to be together."

"So, Melissa, when did you take the overdose?"

"Day before yesterday."

"And were you intending to kill yourself when you took the Tylenol?"

"Oh, yeah," she says. "I'd been planning it for a week. I went to Walgreen's three days ago to buy a whole bottle of the Extra Strength. I took about half of it."

"And where were you when this happened?"

"I was in our apartment."

"Anyone else there at the time?"

"No, Scott was out late working. So I took the pills about nine o'clock and went to bed. I felt so serene, so at peace with my decision. I fell asleep. About two o'clock, I got up sick as a dog. I went to the bathroom and started vomiting. I was up for a couple hours. It woke Scott up—he was mad—and he asked me what was wrong. I told him I had the stomach flu. 'Musta been somethin' I ate' were my exact words."

"And why didn't you tell him you had taken an overdose?"

"I didn't want him to take me to the hospital—that's how bad I wanted to die. I had read about taking Tylenol—that it was an effective way to kill yourself, but that it sometimes took up to two days. I figured I could hide it that long—just say I was sick and stay home until I died."

"Then what happened?"

"Well, I kept throwing up. And then I fell into a deep sleep. Scott got nervous and tried to wake me up. He couldn't, so he called an ambulance." Melissa Peters weeps into her nightgown. "I don't really want to die." Her mother comforts her, holding her daughter's hand, murmuring reassurances into her ear.

"Now look what you done!" says Scott. "I'm getting out of here for a little while—before I get too mad."

"Okay," I say softly into space.

I walk to the other side of the bed and bend down, putting my hand on Melissa's shoulder. "I'm sorry you're having such a hard time," I say.

She looks at me and says quietly, "Me, too. I don't want to die. Look at how it's hurt my mom, and my fiancé. This is awful."

"Well, as a precaution, I'm going to continue the 5150 hold for now. You won't be able to leave the hospital, and I might extend it for you to be transferred to the psych ward when all of this medical stuff clears up. Are you getting any therapy out in Modesto these days?"

"Yes."

"Are you on any psych meds."

"Well, I was, but my AA sponsor told me I better go off them, so I can live a 100 percent clean-and-sober life."

"You go to AA?" I ask.

"Oh, yeah, it's my lifeline. I've been clean and sober for just over six months now. I am powerless over alcohol and drugs. I am an alcoholic and a pill addict. I can say that now."

"Did the psych meds help?"

"Yeah, I was on Zoloft—it helped a lot. My moods were more even. I wasn't getting so angry all the time."

"Is it okay if I give your therapist a call—let her know a bit about what's going on, and she can tell me what you guys have been dealing with in therapy?"

"Yes. Her name is Christy Mathewson, and I forget her phone number."

"No worries. The number's in the chart. I'll give her a call. I will be back tomorrow. And I will touch base with the rest of the liver team. Let's all hope your liver recovers and you don't need a transplant. Now that would be good news!" I am reassuring myself as much as Melissa or her mother.

"Yes, it would, doctor. I'll see you tomorrow."

The clinical psychologist Christy Mathewson returns my call about two hours later—perfect timing, an hour before the liver transplant team meeting is set to begin. "Oh, my God, Dr. Linde," she begins, "the problem is that boyfriend. He's probably dealing drugs. He says he's quit the gang that he was in as an adolescent, but I'm not sure. I don't think he hits her, but I know they have some awful screaming matches."

"How about her mother? Is she a solid person?"

"Well, it depends on what you mean by 'solid.' If you mean, is her house paid for, is her retirement payment sufficient, and is she reliable with appointments and things like that, then I'd say she's solid. She is a good, kindhearted person, but she's been too passive and too goddamn enabling when it comes to her husbands and boyfriends. She's well meaning but chronically overwhelmed—frankly, depressed. I think she should be on meds."

"So what is your working diagnosis of Melissa? Do you think she's a borderline?"

"Is the pope Catholic?" answers Dr. Mathewson. "I'm not much for labels, they don't really inform the therapeutic work, but yes, she has borderline personality, recurrent major depression, alcohol dependence, in remission."

"So, it's true, she is sober these days?"

"Yeah, it's kind of miraculous, I'd say. One day she just came in and said, 'I'm tired of this shit, I can't take the hangovers. I don't like what it does to me. I want to quit.' So I referred her to AA, and she really took to the meetings. She can quote the Big Book chapter and verse, and she's working the twelve steps. I think she's on step four."

"Maybe that's what precipitated her suicide attempt," I muse, knowing that the "ruthless" personal inventory has driven many other patients of mine back to drinking or worse.

"Yeah," says Dr. Mathewson with a knowing laugh. "You know, Dr. Linde, Melissa Peters has a lot of potential. She had a rocky start. Her father left home when she was three. Mom has had a steady string of loser husbands and boyfriends—thankfully none now. I've suspected all along that Melissa may have been the victim of molestation by one of those shiftless good-for-nothings. Melissa denies it, not vehemently, mind you, but if indeed she has been abused, she's not ready to tackle those issues just yet."

"Has she ever talked about suicide with you?"

"Well, she was admitted with that vertical wrist cut, but in reviewing the action with her, the cutting sounded very impulsive. Like a lot of depressed borderlines, she does think frequently about death, but the suicidal thoughts are passive. She is a bit of a risk taker—I mean, look at her boyfriend—and she does often say that she wishes she had never been born." Dr. Mathewson pauses, and then asks, "Is she going to make it medically?"

"I hope so, but it's too early to tell. The numbers on her liver function tests keep rising, so we'll have to take it day by day. She may require a liver transplant if her liver fails."

"Well, heaven help her," she says.

"No kidding."

. . .

The transplant team meets once a week for about two hours. Among other things, we discuss new candidates. In addition to the liver specialists and surgeons, the team includes several nurse-specialists, two social workers, a psychiatrist, and a registered dietician.

Many candidates are highly motivated, with solid long-term recovery from alcohol and drugs, excellent social supports, and a good track record of compliance. No controversies there. A few candidates end up losing out on the opportunity for a transplant by relapsing hard into alcohol or drug consumption or by missing appointment after appointment without reasonable excuses. And, of course, there are a fair number of folks sitting somewhere in between. Perhaps everything about a candidate's case looks strong except for the social supports. Or the candidate has missed a couple of appointments among many. Ambivalence can literally be a killer here.

The greatest challenges for the transplant team lie in predicting ongoing abstinence from drugs and alcohol and in dealing with personality-disordered individuals. You can't, of course, deny an organ to someone because you don't like him or her. But you can deny an organ transplant if you think a person is unlikely to work collaboratively with the team and comply with treatment protocols. Having a psychiatric illness does not necessarily work against a person being evaluated for an organ transplant. "Psychiatric conditions, if well-controlled, do not obviate transplant candidacy," one psychiatrist notes. The only absolute psychiatric contraindications to receiving a liver via transplant are "severe mental retardation, dementia, active suicidality, and intractable noncompliance." At most transplant centers, active alcohol or drug use is also an absolute contraindication.[5]

Being identified as a high or very high risk, from a psychiatric standpoint, generally precludes a person from receiving an organ. In other words, such a person is never even listed as a candidate for transplant. Someone with a moderate or moderately high risk will often be listed with the stipulation that he or she must maintain ongoing abstinence from alcohol and drugs, as documented by random urine toxicological tests, as well as near-perfect compliance with recommendations by the liver team. These may run the gamut from attendance at a certain number of AA meetings per week, to visits to a therapist or a psychiatrist (or both), to evaluations by other specialists, to regular appointments with his or her primary care doctor and liver specialist.

Because Melissa Peters has just arrived in the hospital as a fulminant, her case is a high priority. The social worker doesn't mince words in describing Scott: "During my assessment, he was irritable and uncooperative. I felt in danger being around him. He feels like a sociopath to me. The mother, on the other hand, was mostly delightful. She seemed like a relatively good support person if she can handle this Scott character. I would say that, from a psychosocial standpoint, Ms. Peters is at least a moderate risk. I'll let Paul talk about the patient's suicide risk."

I sigh before I begin. "Well, it's kind of a mixed bag here. I found some encouraging things, some not so encouraging things. I interviewed the patient in the presence of her mother and boyfriend. I also had a chance to talk with the patient's psychologist, who was very helpful. As you know, Ms. Peters is a twenty-four-year-old single Euro-American woman from Modesto who was admitted late last night for a Tylenol overdose. The overdose was intentional, and she tried to hide it from her boyfriend—at a time when early intervention might have prevented her liver injury. It was almost twenty-four hours later that she went to the hospital. She was placed on a 5150. She does have a history of at least one previous suicide attempt by wrist cutting. She is chronically passively suicidal and has a long history of self-injury, though she hasn't engaged in this behavior in about a year. She has a history of alcohol dependence and has been sober by all reports for about six months. She also apparently has an unspecified history of prescription pill addiction.

She is in therapy and has gotten better, but she's gone off her antidepressant, Zoloft, and seems to have worsened since then. It's not really clear what's going on with the boyfriend, but I agree that he is a negative influence. It seems, though, with all of her abandonment issues and probable borderline personality, she will remain attached to him, mostly because she is terrified of being alone. Too bad she didn't pick a nicer guy." Murmurs and laughter spread around the table at that one. "Her diagnoses are recurrent major depression, alcohol abuse in remission, unspecified prescription pill dependence, and probable borderline personality disorder. I would say her acute suicide risk is low to moderate. I am continuing the 5150 for now, though I don't anticipate that she'll need to be admitted to the inpatient psychiatric ward if she stabilizes medically. I would put her risk for transplant in the moderate range from a psychiatric standpoint."

The surgeon, who has been listening intently, speaks first. "She seems emotionally unstable to me. And her boyfriend what an asshole. How do we know she's not gonna get addicted to pain pills, relapse on alcohol, and try and kill herself again? I hate to use a liver for someone who might just blow it out in a year or so."

Dr. Sokol then asks the surgeon, "Do you think she's not a candidate then?"

"Well," the veteran surgeon says, hedging, "I don't think she's a very good candidate. If the team feels like she can make it and work with us, then I'll go ahead. But I do have reservations."

The social worker speaks up: "She's really borderline, Paul. I've heard already from the nursing staff that she's pitting nurses against each other—idealizing some and devaluing others. And, of course, that boyfriend is driving all of them nuts. He hasn't actually threatened anyone or hit anyone, but I think everyone in the unit is afraid of him."

"Of course, we can hope that her numbers come back and she doesn't need a transplant, but we do need to come to a decision today," says Dr. Sokol. "I think we'll really have to leave it up to Paul. Paul, what do you think?"

"Bob, in this case, I would probably err on the side of saying it's worth the psychiatric risk to list her for a transplant. On the plus side, the therapist who is working with her seems very motivated and sharp. Melissa has been showing up for all of her weekly appointments. Her personality disorder seems to be relatively contained by it. She has a history of a good response to Zoloft— we can make it a precondition for her getting listed: that she keeps going to therapy and AA meetings and restarts the Zoloft. She will have a chronic suicide risk higher than the average person, but I think her risk profile really improves when she doesn't drink, goes to therapy regularly, and takes her antidepressant."

"And dumps the boyfriend," says the social worker.

"We can't control who people choose to be associated with," I say. "Maybe she'll pull her act together with the help of the therapist and break up with him. But we can't deny her a liver because we don't like her, and we especially can't just because we don't like her boyfriend. I think the mother is solid enough to help her daughter through this. I would err on the side of advocating for her on the basis of our ability to mitigate her long-term suicidal risk by mandating those changes."

"Okay, team, let's list her, with critical status, as of the end of this meeting," says Dr. Sokol. "But let's hope she won't need a new liver."

We are on the brink of moving on to discuss the next patient when the surgeon clears his throat and speaks. "I'm sorry, Bob, but I'm going to have to veto this one. I see this patient as someone who is unlikely to be compliant with her posttransplant care and is at a high risk of relapsing on alcohol or drugs when the going gets rough. I will have to defer to Paul on the patient's suicide risk, but I've seen too many cases like this go wrong in the long run. I appreciate Paul's evaluation and advocacy, but I just see her as too big of a risk to take care of a new liver."

Though it does seem harsh to me at the time, in fairness to the surgeon he isn't making this decision in a vacuum. Research from both the medical and psychiatric literature around this time indicate suboptimal outcomes with transplants for patients with fulminant hepatic failure, less than six months of sobriety and depression, and/or a personality disorder.[6]

"All right, team," says Bob. "Though we work as a team, as the surgeon you do have the right and responsibility to veto as you see fit. We won't list her. And we'll hope for the best. If her numbers keep bumping up, then we'll have to inform her and the family that we don't think she is a candidate."

.   .   .

I arrive on the unit the next morning. Apparently Melissa had a difficult night. She got disoriented and confused, and it appears that the boyfriend panicked and flew out of there. She has likely endured a bout of delirium, which is no surprise, given the gravity of her medical illness. To reduce her agitation, she was given some intravenous Haldol and Ativan and was seen by the psychiatric resident on call, who wrote a brief note about it.

I notice in the lab section that the numbers from her liver function tests continue to rise. My heart sinks. I know these things can fluctuate, but I also know that she is receiving state-of-the-art, optimal, aggressive medical treatment for a Tylenol overdose. Her other labs look okay, but I notice a slight worsening of her kidney function test results.

I step into the room and see that Melissa is sleeping. Her mother is dozing in a chair. "Good morning, Mrs. Peters." She awakens, startled.

"Sorry, doctor, I didn't get much sleep last night."

"Yeah, I heard it was a rough night. What happened?"

"Well, it started out okay. She finally fell asleep about eleven thirty. They gave her a sleeping pill, but I knew she was pretty exhausted. After she dozed off, then I went to sleep in this recliner here. But I was awakened by her shouting at about two. She was screaming, 'Mother, get them out of here. Those machines, they've turned into monsters, they're telling me that they're gonna kill me.'

"'What machines, honey?' I asked.

"'Those!' she screamed. She pointed to the cardiac and respiratory monitor, the IV poles on either side of her bed, and at the TV over her head there. She said the machines had mutated into monsters and were now tearing, stabbing, grinding, and punching at her."

"Then what happened?"

"Well, the nurse heard the screams, of course, and the two of us were able to get her calmed down enough, though she kept talking about the monsters. I think the nurse gave her some medications in her IV and she went back to sleep. But she was up again at three thirty and again at five thirty. Poor baby, she is totally pooped out. Doctor, you're the psychiatrist. Do you think she's having a nervous breakdown—all the stress?"

"That's a good question. Stress sure doesn't help. But what you observed was delirium, a change in behavior that is yet another complication of her medical illness. As I'm sure you know, the brain as an organ depends on a steady supply of oxygen and blood sugar and a set of normal or nearly normal lab values to function properly. What you observed likely was caused by abnormal labs or was a side effect of one of the medications she received. The good news here is that delirium gets better on its own, and we help it along by reviewing her medication list, correcting her labs, giving her a bit of medication as necessary."

"Speaking of which," says Mrs. Peters, "Dr. Sokol told me some bad news this morning."

"What?" I ask, as nonchalantly as I can. I am acutely aware of the really bad news that Melissa won't be able to get a new liver if the Tylenol overdose nukes her original one.

"He said the liver numbers were rising, but he said they often see that kind of pattern in this kind of overdose."

Well, he's the liver specialist, I think. "Yeah, we're all just kind of in a wait-and-watch holding pattern. The uncertainty is very hard to deal with," I say, speaking at the time for both of us. "Are you religious, Mrs. Peters?"

"Yes, we're Episcopalian. Our pastor, our church, and our family and friends are praying for us right now."

"I imagine that that gives you some reassurance, some peace of mind."

"Yes, doctor, thank you for asking."

"Sure. I'm going to let Melissa sleep for now. I will stop in early tomorrow morning."

"You mean at six o'clock, with the rest of the team?"

"No, I meant more like eight thirty. We psychiatrists keep banker's hours compared to those rock stars of medicine."

. . .

The next day I pick up her chart and start flipping toward the labs. Her AST is 14,000, up from 12,500 yesterday. Oh, shit, I think. Her liver is going to buy it, and she's going to die without a new one. I see Melissa's mom walking down the hallway, and I get up to say hi.

"How are things this morning?"

"Well, she slept more last night, but her nausea and vomiting seem to be on the upswing. They also tell me she's at an increased risk of bleeding. I don't quite understand it."

"Hmm, what do the liver doctors have to say about it?"

"They say not to worry; we're not out of the woods yet, but that she's doing about as expected. I asked them about the possibility of a transplant if her liver fails."

"And what did they say?"

"To cross that bridge when we come to it. They don't think Melissa is going to need it, so I have to trust them."

I gulp. I don't know if Mrs. Peters knows about the rising liver function numbers. Melissa still needs to be in the unit. She is finishing her course of intravenous medicine and still needs to be monitored closely.

"Any word from Scott?"

"No, he's still missing in action. You know, doctor, Melissa may not want to hear this from me, but I hope this episode drives Scott away. He's been a bad influence on her. The irony in all of this is that, with this overdose, she was trying to draw him closer—to make him realize just how much she needed him. Forgive me for saying this, but he's a rat."

"You're entitled to your opinion, Mrs. Peters," I say as neutrally as I can, though I think she may be on to something. "Is she awake now?"

"Yes."

I knock on the door and make my way in. A nurse is adjusting one of the IV poles. Melissa lies still on the bed.

"How are you doing?" I start.

She sighs deeply. "Oh, all right, I guess. I'm really tired. But I am glad I didn't die. What a stupid thing for me to do! I was just so angry at the time, I guess, mostly at Scott for not being around when I needed him."

"What's your sense of why you took so many pills? What was it—half a bottle of Extra Strength Tylenol? Clearly enough to be fatal."

"Oh, God, I wasn't thinking about that, I wasn't thinking about anything. My mind was a blank; I was blinded by fury. I just kept taking them by the handful, one after the other."

"But you ended up hurting yourself the most."

"It's lucky I didn't take the entire bottle—then, I understand, I wouldn't have any chance of living without getting a liver transplant."

I cringe again. Even though I was the one who had advocated a transplant for her, I still feel some guilt at the team's rejecting her. "Have the doctors talked to you at all about whether you might need a transplant?"

"Well, not since the first day. I guess we're all just hoping I don't need one. But if I have to go through all that, then I'm prepared to do what needs to be done."

"Do you still feel you're at risk of killing yourself?"

"Well, not in the foreseeable future. It's something that my therapist and I have talked a lot about. Because of my abuse history, I feel a need to maintain some control. And killing yourself is the ultimate in control. And I am more depressed than ever."

"Why is that, do you think?"

"Well, a lot of it is my fucked-up relationship. Like, Scott bolted day before yesterday and hasn't been heard from since. Knowing him, he'll show up later today or tomorrow with a big bouquet of flowers and some story of why it took him two days to come back. I think I'm going to have to break up with him." She starts crying. "At least it would make my mom happy." She cries harder. "I don't know how Scott will take it. He can be awfully jealous."

"I'm sorry this is such a struggle for you."

"Yeah, me too." She pauses. "I guess the silver lining in all of this is that, although I'm incredibly tired, I am seeing things a little more clearly. How I can live without Scott. Sure, it's gonna hurt, but I have my mom, I have some good friends, I have my AA sponsor."

Melissa struggles to keep her eyes open.

"Hey, I'll let you sleep now. Hope you feel better. And I'll come and see you tomorrow."

She doesn't answer. She is fast asleep. I have enough information that I can drop Melissa's psychiatric hold and not subject her to our local psych ward. That is good news, which I'll have to relay to her tomorrow.

.   .   .

The next day I go to the unit once again. I am surprised to discover that Melissa Peters isn't there anymore. My heart sinks. Does this mean she's dead? I find her regular nurse, whom I recognize from previous days, and reluctantly approach her.

"Hi, I'm Dr. Linde, the liver psychiatrist."

"Hi."

"It's about Melissa Peters. Has she . . . has she . . ." I stammer.

"Has she been transferred to the floor?" asks the nurse, clearly in a hurry. "Yes, earlier this morning. She's on Five East."

"Thank you, thank you."

I stop in the doctor's lounge and look up Melissa's labs on the computer. Sweet! Her AST is below 10,000 and her other labs are normalizing. She is now very unlikely to need a transplant. Whew!

I go down to Five East and find her room. I go in. An older man and two young women are standing near Doreen Peters.

"Hi, doctor," says Doreen, smiling. "I'd like you to meet some very important people in Melissa's life. This is my father, her grandfather Joshua. And these two pretty young ladies are Sara and Tricia, two of Melissa's oldest and dearest friends."

"Pleased to meet you. I'm Dr. Linde, the psychiatrist for the liver team," I say, shaking hands all around.

I turn my attention to Melissa, whose color is returning to normal. She is much more alert.

"How are you doing today?"

"Just great. I heard my labs are improving. I feel better; I guess I won't need the transplant."

"And I have some more good news. You won't need to be transferred to a locked psychiatric unit after your stay here."

She looks grateful. "Thank God." She pauses before saying, "You mean you don't think I'm crazy?"

I pause the requisite period of time before responding, "Well, I never said *that*."

Her friends burst out laughing, and Melissa joins them.

"Listen, Melissa, I've been doing this work for more than ten years now, and I've seen literally thousands of psychotic patients, so I know crazy. And you, young lady, are not crazy. Stressed, depressed, in recovery? Sure. But crazy? No."

"Well, that's a relief," says her mother earnestly, invoking another round of chuckles throughout the whole room.

"I've been talking to your therapist, Melissa, and we agree that you could benefit from a very specific group treatment for borderline personality disorder called DBT, which stands for 'dialectical behavioral therapy.' This would be in addition to your regular therapy, getting back on Zoloft, and staying sober. Dr. Mathewson told me that a new DBT group is starting up at a community clinic near your house."

"Well, tell Dr. Mathewson to sign me up!" she says.

"I will, I will. It should help you a lot. It's really practical and gives you some tools for dealing with other people."

"Sounds good. I could use some," she laughs. "Thank you for your help."

"I will leave you to your guests, Melissa, and check in with you again tomorrow. Congratulations!"

"Thank you, doctor."

"Pleased to have met all of you," I say before leaving.

STRAIGHT FROM THE HEART

We work in the dark—we do what we can—we give what we have.
Our doubt is our passion and our passion is our task. The rest is the
madness of art.

Henry James, *The Middle Years*

As an emergency psychiatrist working on the front line, I have the task of putting a human face on the system, on the institution, of mitigating the legal, financial, political, and bureaucratic constraints that we, both patient and professional, find ourselves in. To accomplish this, I must work with not my best *face* forward, but my best *heart* forward. How does one do this?

Now that I've offered seventy thousand or so words in this book as a psychiatrist and a writer, with as much or more left on the cutting-room floor, I am wondering about the wisdom of trying to explain in words what it's like, or more literally what it has *felt* like, to be an emergency psychiatrist. How do I reconcile two very different experiences of being a psychiatrist—one represented by the head and words, the other symbolized by the heart and emotions?

233

To me as a writer, words are currency. To me as a physician, too, and particularly as a psychiatrist, words are currency, and they will continue to be important in my life. Their meaning and significance, however, must always be considered in a context. Words are powerful, but they are not the *real things*. They are representatives, proxies, pointers, and indicators. A single word cannot, in and of itself, be the *thing*.

Things are held nonverbally, in unbound immaterial realms—beyond words—in the heart, the soul, the spirit. Emotions transcend words. They are to be experienced and considered—to be *felt*. And it is in the language of feelings where authentic healing begins—for both doctor and patient.

While I cannot fail to recognize and address painful emotions in my patients and my self, it is also my task to seek energetic joy and humor in the moment, to experience the buzz of empathy. This *is* the reward to be found in the work.

The author C. S. Lewis describes the beneficial reciprocity of altruism in his book *Mere Christianity,* which could have just as easily been called *Mere Empathy.* Empathy causes a rush. It's addictive. Recent advances in the neurosciences confirm that the experience of deep empathy, with its associated glow of euphoria, shares some final common neurobiological pleasure pathways with narcotics, alcohol, and cigarettes. In other words, empathy is addictive and pleasurable.[1]

How can you maintain a sense of humor, sanity, and compassion and an empathetic stance in a place like psych emergency, where nearly impossible challenges present themselves every day? The most adaptive way to deal with all the stress is to focus on the present moment, on the task at hand, and on the human being sitting across from you in the interview room, whose needs and concerns should be your primary interest. Tune in and address your colleagues and patients in the present moment: connect, rehumanize yourself, do what you can, give what you have.

William Carlos Williams describes his experience of engaging deeply with patients: "I lost myself in the very properties of their minds: for the moment at least I actually became them, whoever they should be, so that when I detached myself from them at the end of a half-hour of intense concentration over some illness which was affecting them, it was as though I was reawakening from a sleep. For the moment I myself did not exist, nothing of myself affected me. As a consequence I came back to myself, as from any other sleep, rested."[2]

I am familiar with that feeling—of being lost in the moment while writing or while working with patients in psych emergency. How can one otherwise get the job done? I know this state of mind is the same pathway reached by anyone deeply absorbed in a task, creative or otherwise. Your ability to access this state of mind provides a powerful pointer to what is most important to you and to the task or tasks in which you feel most at home.

How does one even approach understanding another person? And, then, how does one begin to describe what he or she has seen or experienced with another person? "The difficulty," writes Williams, "is to catch the evasive life of the thing, to phrase the words in such a way that stereotype will yield a moment of insight. That is where the difficulty lies. We are lucky when that underground current can be tapped and the secret spring of all our lives will send up its pure water. It seldom happens. . . . Do we not see that we are inarticulate? That is what defeats us. It is our inability to communicate to another how we are locked within ourselves, unable to say the simplest thing of importance to one another, any of us, even the most valuable, that makes our lives like those of a litter of kittens in a wood-pile. That gives the physician, and I don't mean the high-priced psychoanalyst, his opportunity; psychoanalysis amounts to no more than another dialectic into which to be locked." Williams puts it this way in describing how physicians listen to patients: "It is that, we realize, which beyond all they have been saying is what they have been trying to say. . . . We begin to see that the underlying meaning of all they want to tell us and have always failed to communicate is the poem. . . . The poem springs from the half-spoken words of such patients as the physician sees from day to day. . . . In that the secret lies. This, in the end, comes perhaps to be the occupation of the physician after a lifetime of careful listening."[3]

The poem is Williams's lovely metaphor for understanding the essence of things in an oblique, indirect manner. He is one of the very few who can truly capture essence with words. This "secret spring" of "pure water" can survive only transiently in a world defined by words. It is accessible to mortals only as an ephemeral glimpse. It is freshest in a nonverbal realm, in a world of feelings, emotions, a world of the heart.

I discovered this: My heart, and not my words, provides the first and strongest line of defense when protecting myself in my work as a psychiatrist. In a seemingly paradoxical way, my best self-protection derives from actually opening my heart and laying its contents bare.

I experienced a measure of serenity and acceptance when I finally felt free enough to admit to myself that, while my head works pretty well, my real strength as a physician comes from the heart.

NOTES

PREFACE

Epigraph: Viktor Frankl was trained as a physician and psychiatrist in the first half of the twentieth century. While this book is understandably well known and acclaimed for Frankl's incredibly moving documentation of his survival in a World War II concentration camp, it also provides an inspiring rebuttal to the era's existential nihilism and collective insanity. With his formation of a school of psychotherapeutic thought, which he called *logotherapy,* he placed an emphasis on an individual finding a sense of meaning and meanings to be fulfilled in the future. It is an action-oriented therapy based on hope despite our living in uncertain times. He carried forth a central mission of rehumanizing not just the practice of psychiatry but also that of clinical medicine as a whole. Quotation from *Man's Search for Meaning* by Viktor E. Frankl. Copyright © 1959, 1962, 1984, 1992 by Viktor E. Frankl. Reprinted by permission of Beacon Press, Boston.

    1. T. M. Luhrmann, *Of Two Minds: An Anthropologist Looks at American Psychiatry* (New York: Vintage, 2001), 119. Tanya Luhrmann is an award-winning author and anthropologist currently on the faculty of Stanford University. In this passage, she directly refers to her observations in acute care psychiatry. She has had a distinguished career in academics, much of it at the University of Chicago. The focus of her work has been on clarifying the multiple interfaces among psychology,

spirituality, and anthropology. This book is an exacting and compre-hensive documentation and analysis of the state of American psychia-try in the late twentieth and early twenty-first centuries. It greatly propelled me forward in my conceptualization of *Danger to Self*.

2. R. Selzer, *The Exact Location of the Soul: New and Selected Essays* (New York: Picador USA, 2001), 219. To put it succinctly, Richard Selzer is the dean of American physician-authors. He enjoyed a long and distinguished career as an academic surgeon at Yale, and he now spends much of his time studying and writing in the medical school library there. He has written some of this era's quintessential essays for students of medicine, which are reprinted in this collection—namely, "Skin," "The Knife," "The Corpse," "Textbook," and "Letter(s) to a Young Surgeon." The passage quoted here is from "Letter to a Young Surgeon I." Selzer's description of a typical (for him) psychiatrist is very much a product of his having undergone medical education and surgical training during a time when Freud was king of psychiatry and psychoanalysts prevailed, especially on the East Coast.

3. P. R. Linde, *Of Spirits and Madness: An American Psychiatrist in Africa* (New York: McGraw-Hill, 2002).

1 THE ER DOC

1. R. D. Laing, *Wisdom, Madness, and Folly: The Making of a Psychiatrist* (New York: McGraw-Hill, 1985), 5–6, emphasis in the original. R. D. Laing was an influential Scottish psychiatrist with a bit of a rebellious streak. He, along with the American psychiatrist Thomas Szasz, author of *The Myth of Mental Illness,* called into ques-tion the psychiatrists of a certain era who enjoyed nearly unquestioned authority in dealing with patients. Libertarians Laing and Szasz, prod-ucts of a progressive era, likely influenced public opinion, judges, leg-islators, and policy makers, who essentially stripped psychiatrists of much of their power. Civil liberties seemed to be enhanced, but the downside was that this gave politicians like California's governor Ronald Reagan an opportunity and the impetus to unfund the care of

a voiceless and often vulnerable population of psychiatrically ill people, and to unhospitalize them under the pretext of freeing them. This marked the beginning of an era in which we added substantially to our nation's homeless population while criminalizing the mentally ill. I'm certain this was not what Laing or Szasz had in mind.

2. B. J. Sadock and V. A. Sadock, eds., *Kaplan and Sadock's Synopsis of Psychiatry* (Lippincott Williams & Wilkins, 2003), 1357. This is one fat synopsis—1,460 pages for the condensed version of the mammoth bible of American psychiatry, customarily known as "Kaplan and Sadock," after the original coeditors. The unabridged version tops out at three volumes and nearly 4,000 pages.

2 THE ROOKIE

1. R. A. MacDonald, *A Country Doctor's Chronicle: Further Tales from the Northwoods* (St. Paul: Minnesota Historical Society, 2004), 29. Roger A. MacDonald is a retired family physician from northern Minnesota. I see his book as a bridge between early-twentieth-century physicians—including the famous, such as William Carlos Williams, and the not-so-famous, such as my grandfather Herman Linde—and me. MacDonald's book, the second in a series, is eminently readable and documents the work of a country doctor in northern wilderness and farm country well before the dawn of the Internet age.

3 THE SCRAMBLER

1. R. I. Simon, *Bad Men Do What Good Men Dream: A Forensic Psychiatrist Illuminates the Darker Side of Human Behavior* (Washington, DC: American Psychiatric Press, 1996), 250. You've got to love the title of this book. Robert Simon, a Harvard professor, is one of the leading forensic psychiatrists in the nation. In clear and entertaining prose, he makes complex issues understandable and makes them come alive.

2. Ibid., 274.

3. M. Gladwell, *Blink: The Power of Thinking without Thinking* (New York: Little, Brown, 2005), 33–34. Malcolm Gladwell, who also writes for the *New Yorker,* has actually made cognitive psychology, information processing technology, and consciousness theory fun, not to mention highly edifying. I read this book in order to study the nascent science of human decision analysis so that I could begin to understand what I always thought was my idiosyncratic approach to clinical decision-making in psych emergency. My usual modus operandi in clinical psychiatry has been to make a provisional decision relatively early during an interview—in particular, a decision on whether to release someone from psych emergency. Then I move backward in my thought process and ask myself questions to sort out what my rationale and logical justifications would have to be if I were to go with that decision. Gladwell's book made me feel much better about my seemingly convoluted way of coming to conclusions.

4. B. J. Sadock and V. A. Sadock, eds., *Kaplan and Sadock's Comprehensive Textbook of Psychiatry,* 8th ed. (Philadelphia: Lippincott Williams & Wilkins, 2005), 3975.

5. Ibid.

6. Gladwell, *Blink,* 12.

7. Ibid., 107.

8. B. J. Sadock and V. A. Sadock, eds., *Kaplan and Sadock's Synopsis of Psychiatry,* 9th ed. (Philadelphia: Lippincott Williams & Wilkins, 2003), 1355.

9. Ibid.

10. Simon, *Bad Men Do What Good Men Dream,* 274–75.

11. J. Monahan et al., "Developing a Clinically Useful Actuarial Tool for Assessing Violence Risk," *British Journal of Psychiatry* 176 (2000): 312–19.

4 THE PSYCHODYNAMO

1. D. S. Viscott, *The Making of a Psychiatrist* (Greenwich, CT: Fawcett Publications, 1973), 129. This was one of the first books I read

when I started working on *Danger to Self.* Written more than three decades ago, in a much different era of psychiatric practice, *The Making of a Psychiatrist* captured many of the cross-generational dilemmas inherent in trying to treat patients with psychiatric illnesses. Viscott's literary voice and tone felt simpatico with mine. This was his first book; he went on to write innumerable self-help books and created a television show in Southern California, before dying prematurely of heart disease in his late fifties.

2. T. Lewis, F. Amini, and R. Lannon, *A General Theory of Love* (New York: Random House, 2000), 186–87. A trio of UCSF psychiatrists collaborated to write this erudite and fascinating book, striving to clarify the background of our complex slate of emotions and the subtleties of the human experience. The first of the three coauthors is one of my contemporaries; the other two were teachers of mine—one (now deceased) was a prominent psychoanalyst, and the other primarily a psychopharmacologist. I read the book with great interest and was especially influenced by its perspective on the biology-psychology split.

3. D. H. Brendel, *Healing Psychiatry: Bridging the Science/Humanism Divide,* foreword by T. M. Luhrmann (Cambridge, MA: MIT Press, 2006), 16. I stumbled across this book relatively late in my writing process. It very much helped me to discover the evidence behind my pragmatic approach to patients, which, of course, I developed mostly organically—in a trial-and-error, feeling-my-way-along, reinventing-the-wheel sort of way. The Harvard psychiatrist David Brendel is a scholar of the highest order—a gifted clinical psychiatrist, respected educator, and, most of all, bioethicist, philosopher, and thinker who has been trying to formally sort out many of the existential, ethical, and even economic quandaries inherent in the modern practice of clinical psychiatry.

4. Lewis, Amini, and Lannon, *A General Theory of Love,* 91.

5. Ibid., 171.

6. T. M. Luhrmann, *Of Two Minds: An Anthropologist Looks at American Psychiatry* (New York: Vintage, 2001), 9.

7. Viscott, *The Making of a Psychiatrist,* 132.

8. Luhrmann, *Of Two Minds,* 7.

9. P. D. Kramer, *Listening to Prozac: The Landmark Book about Antidepressants and the Remaking of the Self* (New York: Penguin, 1997), 6, 20, 331. Outside of perhaps a self-help author or two, Peter Kramer is likely the nation's most famous psychiatrist-writer. He is best known for capturing the zeitgeist of the 1990s with *Listening to Prozac,* but he has also written a regular column for a psychiatric industry newspaper, as well as several other books, including a novel. He is indeed one of the brightest minds of modern American psychiatry. In this book, Kramer fully captures the dilemmas involved in trying to stake out the middle ground of psychiatry, between psychology and biology. With *Listening to Prozac,* he opened a door for investigative journalists who would take a closer look at the day-to-day practices of the monstrously profitable pharmaceutical industry. But most of all, he is a master clinician, as demonstrated in the stories he tells of his patient encounters. He is an important role model for an entire generation of psychiatrists.

5 THE JAILER

1. H. Shinichiro et al., "2-Nonenal Newly Found in Human Body Odor Tends to Increase with Aging," *Journal of Investigative Dermatology* 116 (2001): 520.
2. R. D. Laing, *Wisdom, Madness, and Folly: The Making of a Psychiatrist* (New York: McGraw-Hill, 1985), 4, 13, 19.
3. T. M. Luhrmann, *Of Two Minds: An Anthropologist Looks at American Psychiatry* (New York: Vintage, 2001), 222–23.
4. J. R. Elpers, "Public Mental Health Funding in California, 1959 to 1989," *Hospital and Community Psychiatry* 40, no. 8 (1989): 799.
5. Luhrmann, *Of Two Minds,* 223.
6. J. Geller, "The Last Half-Century of Psychiatric Services as Reflected in Psychiatric Services," *Psychiatric Services* 51, no. 1 (January 2000): 42.
7. B. J. Sadock and V. A. Sadock, eds., *Kaplan and Sadock's Synopsis of Psychiatry,* 9th ed. (Philadelphia: Lippincott Williams & Wilkins, 2003), 1357.

8. APA Task Force on Psychiatric Emergency Services, "The Expert Consensus Guide Series: Treatment of Behavioral Emergencies," American Association of Emergency Psychiatry, www .emergencypsychiatry.org, accessed March 20, 2009.

6 THE JURY

1. R. D. Ellenhorn, *Parasuicidality and Paradox: Breaking through the Medical Model* (New York: Springer, 2008), xiv. The sociologist, social worker, and psychotherapist Ross D. Ellenhorn puts a very different spin on the problem of chronically suicidal and manipulative recidivistic patients, who monopolize a disproportionate amount of the time and energy of those who work in hospitals and clinics and whose treatment consumes a disproportionate quantity of the funding available for mental health services.

2. Ibid., xiv, xiii.

3. C. Towle, *Common Human Needs* (1945; reprint, Silver Spring, MD: National Association of Social Workers, 1987), xxii. I can thank my father for pointing me to this book, which he said was a mainstay of social work training in the 1950s, when he did his graduate work at Indiana University. When read in the context of the audience for which it was intended—namely, benefits workers staffing the front lines of social welfare offices after World War II—the book does not strike one as being in any way controversial. But as read by McCarthy-era witch-hunters, this book appeared to be nothing less than a full-scale attack on the American way of life.

4. T. Dalrymple, *Life at the Bottom: The Worldview That Makes the Underclass* (Chicago: Ivan R. Dee Books, 2001), 132–33, 182–83. Theodore Dalrymple is a culturally conservative pseudonymous British libertarian psychiatrist who, via books like this one and a regular column in the conservative newspapers *London Spectator* and *City Journal,* throws red meat to right-wing ideologues. Nonetheless, he does make some astute observations about what now seems to be a perpetual underclass. He dares to ask difficult and controversial questions

about whether the welfare state is really helping people or slowly making things worse. His work is always thought-provoking and sometimes just provoking.

5. American Psychiatric Association, *Diagnostic and Statistical Manual of Mental Disorders,* 4th ed., text revision (DSM-IV-TR) (Washington, DC: American Psychiatric Association, 2000), 689. This book, a cash cow for organized psychiatry, is just the latest in a series of diagnostic and statistical manuals that attempt to make psychiatric diagnoses more scientific. I will give the book and its system of diagnosis this much credit: it is fairly readable and easy to understand, and its diagnostic guidelines are readily applicable. But the bigger questions are: Does it represent patients in a nuanced, multidimensional fashion that acknowledges the complexity of human experience? And how good can it be if each edition is written and formulated by committees of dozens of psychiatrists?

6. B. J. Sadock and V. A. Sadock, eds., *Kaplan and Sadock's Synopsis of Psychiatry,* 9th ed. (Philadelphia: Lippincott Williams & Wilkins, 2003), 897.

7. DSM-IV-TR, 739, 706.

8. Sadock and Sadock, *Kaplan and Sadock's Synopsis of Psychiatry,* 249.

9. Dalrymple, *Life at the Bottom,* 38.

7 THE CLAIRVOYANT

1. K. R. Jamison, *An Unquiet Mind: A Memoir of Moods and Madness* (New York: Vintage, 1996), 110, 111, 115, 115–16. This book by the noted author and accomplished academic psychologist Kay Redfield Jamison tells the painful and poignant story of her struggle with severe bipolar disorder. A professor of psychiatry at Johns Hopkins, Jamison expertly blends the personal and professional, weaving academic material into her account in a way that does not obscure the riveting details of her life story. The book reflects a remarkable openness and courage.

2. A. D. Taylor, "By My Own Hand," *Bellevue Literary Review* 6, no. 2 (Fall 2006): 120–21. The *Bellevue Literary Review* is a state-of-the-art

literary journal published by members of the medical school faculty of New York University. Its editors periodically devote an entire issue to mental health matters. Taylor eloquently describes the way in which many, many chronically ill individuals think about suicide.

3. S. C. Shea, *The Practical Art of Suicide Assessment: A Guide for Mental Health Professionals and Substance Abuse Counselors* (Hoboken, NJ: John Wiley & Sons, 2002), 13. Psychiatrist Shawn Shea wrote this highly readable book, which includes many illuminating case examples, in an effort to make the assessment of suicide risk more systematic. He does an especially good job of teasing out risk variables that can be discovered only by means of thorough and considered interviewing.

4. Ibid., 153–62.

5. Ibid., 162–77.

6. Ibid., 177–80.

7. Ibid., 180–88.

8 THE SPEED COP

1. Lyrics to "I Need a Miracle" by John Barlow, copyright Ice Nine Publishing Company. Used with permission. From Grateful Dead, *Shakedown Street* (Arista Records/RCA Music Group/Sony BMG, 1978).

2. N. Rasmussen, "Making the First Antidepressant: Amphetamine in American Medicine, 1929–1950," *Journal of the History of Medical and Allied Sciences* 61, no. 3 (2006): 288–323.

3. DanceSafe, "Drug Info," www.dancesafe.org, accessed March 24, 2009. DanceSafe is a nonprofit harm-reduction organization with local chapters throughout the United States and Canada.

4. Tweaker.org, "Crystal 101: Ways Guys Do Meth," www.tweaker .org, accessed March 24, 2009. This is the outreach and educational Web site of the Stonewall Project, a harm-reduction substance abuse treatment clinic for gay and bisexual men who use methamphetamine, located in San Francisco.

5. V. E. Frankl, *Man's Search for Meaning* (1959; reprint, New York: Pocket Books, 1984), 86 87.

6. P. Byrnes, *New Yorker* (August 22, 2005): 58.

7. K. Scott, *SoMa* (New York: Kensington Books, 2007), 261.

8. Frankl, *Man's Search for Meaning,* 99.

9. DSM-IV-TR, 467.

10. M. Isaac and P. Chand, "Dissociative and Conversion Disorders: Defining Boundaries," *Current Opinion in Psychiatry* 19, no. 1 (2006): 61.

9 THE WITNESS

1. J. D. Rouse, "Borderline and Other Dramatic Personality Disorders in the Psychiatric Emergency Service," *Psychiatric Annals* 24, no. 11 (1994): 600. This issue is devoted to the discipline of emergency psychiatry. Dr. Rouse has been a colleague of mine at San Francisco General Hospital since I started my work in psych emergency. He is a master at handling deeply regressed patients in this setting.

2. Ibid.

3. J. A. Schumm, M. Briggs-Phillips, and S. E. Hobfoll, "Cumulative Interpersonal Traumas and Social Support as Risk and Resiliency Factors in Predicting PTSD and Depression among Inner-City Women," *Journal of Traumatic Stress* 19, no. 6 (2006): 825.

4. D. Katerndahl, S. Burge, and N. Kellogg, "Predictors of Development of Adult Psychopathology in Female Victims of Childhood Sexual Abuse," *Journal of Nervous and Mental Disease* 193, no. 4 (2005): 258.

5. E. A. Hoge, E. D. Austin, and M. H. Pollack, "Resilience: Research Evidence and Conceptual Considerations for Posttraumatic Stress Disorder," *Depression and Anxiety* 24, no. 2 (2007): 139.

6. Ibid., 147.

10 THE JUDGE

1. O. Surman, "Psychiatric Aspects of Liver Transplantation," *Psychosomatics* 35, no. 3 (1994): 300.

2. A. L. Caplan and D. H. Coelho, eds., *The Ethics of Organ Transplants: The Current Debate* (Amherst, NY: Prometheus Books, 1998), 249.

3. Ibid., 276.

4. M. Mayhew, "A Review of Acetaminophen Overdose," *Journal for Nurse Practitioners* 3, no. 3 (2007): 186–88.

5. Surman, "Psychiatric Aspects of Liver Transplantation," 301.

6. Caplan and Coelho, *Ethics of Organ Transplants,* 255; R. Osorio et al., "Predicting Recidivism after Orthotopic Liver Transplantation for Alcoholic Liver Disease," *Hepatology* (July 1994): 105; R. C. Chacko et al., "Relationship of Psychiatric Morbidity and Psychosocial Factors in Organ Transplant," *Psychosomatics* 37, no. 2 (March–April 1996): 102.

EPILOGUE

1. P. L. Jackson, E. Brunet, A. N. Meltzoff, and J. Decety, "Empathy Examined through the Neural Mechanisms Involved in Imagining How I Feel versus How You Feel Pain," *Neuropsychologia* 44, no. 5 (2006): 752.

2. W. C. Williams, *The Autobiography of William Carlos Williams* (New York: New Directions, 1951), 356.

3. Ibid., 359, 361, 362.

REFERENCES

American Psychiatric Association. *Diagnostic and Statistical Manual of Mental Disorders*. 4th edition, text revision (DSM-IV-TR). Washington, DC: American Psychiatric Association, 2000.

Appelbaum, P. S. "Ambivalence Codified: California's New Outpatient Commitment Structure." *Psychiatric Services* 54 (2003): 26–28.

Brendel, D. H. *Healing Psychiatry: Bridging the Science/Humanism Divide*. Foreword by T. M. Luhrmann. Cambridge, MA: MIT Press, 2006.

Buckley, R. Audiotaped interview by author, October 2006, Sebastopol, CA.

Burroughs, A. *Running with Scissors*. New York: Picador, 2002.

Byrnes, P. *New Yorker* (August 22, 2005): 58.

Campos, R. "'The Medical Humanities,' for Lack of a Better Term." *JAMA* 294, no. 9 (2005): 1009–11.

Caplan, A. L., and D. H. Coelho, eds. *The Ethics of Organ Transplants: The Current Debate*. Amherst, NY: Prometheus Books, 1998.

Chacko, R. C., et al. "Relationship of Psychiatric Morbidity and Psychosocial Factors in Organ Transplant." *Psychosomatics* 37, no. 2 (March–April 1996): 100–107.

Dalrymple, T. *Life at the Bottom: The Worldview That Makes the Underclass*. Chicago: Ivan R. Dee Books, 2001.

Durkheim, E. *Suicide: A Study in Sociology*. New York: Free Press, 1959

Ellenhorn, R. D. *Parasuicidality and Paradox: Breaking through the Medical Model.* New York: Springer, 2008.

Elpers, J. R. "Public Mental Health Funding in California, 1959 to 1989." *Hospital and Community Psychiatry* 40, no. 8 (1989): 799–804.

Frankl, V. E. *Man's Search for Meaning.* 1959. Reprint, New York: Pocket Books, 1984.

Frey, J. *A Million Little Pieces.* New York: Nan A. Talese/Doubleday, 2003.

———. *My Friend Leonard.* New York: Riverhead Books, 2005.

Gawande, A. *Better: A Surgeon's Notes on Performance.* New York: Picador, 2007.

Geller, J. "The Last Half-Century of Psychiatric Services as Reflected in Psychiatric Services." *Psychiatric Services* 51, no. 1 (January 2000): 41–67.

Gladwell, M. *Blink: The Power of Thinking without Thinking.* New York: Little, Brown, 2005.

Groopman, J. *How Doctors Think.* Boston: Houghton Mifflin, 2007.

Hoge, E. A., E. D. Austin, and M. H. Pollack. "Resilience: Research Evidence and Conceptual Considerations for Posttraumatic Stress Disorder." *Depression and Anxiety* 24, no. 2 (2007): 139–52.

Isaac, M., and P. Chand. "Dissociative and Conversion Disorders: Defining Boundaries." *Current Opinion in Psychiatry* 19, no. 1 (2006): 61–66.

Jackson, P. L., E. Brunet, A. N. Meltzoff, and J. Decety. "Empathy Examined through the Neural Mechanisms Involved in Imagining How I Feel versus How You Feel Pain." *Neuropsychologia* 44, no. 5 (2006): 752–61.

Jamison, K. R. *Night Falls Fast: Understanding Suicide.* New York: Vintage, 2000.

———. *An Unquiet Mind: A Memoir of Moods and Madness.* New York: Vintage, 1996.

Katerndahl, D., S. Burge, and N. Kellogg. "Predictors of Development of Adult Psychopathology in Female Victims of Childhood Sexual Abuse." *Journal of Nervous and Mental Disease* 193, no. 4 (2005): 258–64.

Kesey, K. *One Flew over the Cuckoo's Nest.* 1962. Reprint, New York: Viking/Penguin Classics, 2003.

Kleinman, A. *The Illness Narratives: Suffering, Healing, and the Human Condition.* New York: Basic Books, 1988.

Kramer, P. D. *Listening to Prozac: The Landmark Book about Antidepressants and the Remaking of the Self.* New York: Penguin, 1997.

Laing, R. D. *Wisdom, Madness, and Folly: The Making of a Psychiatrist.* New York: McGraw-Hill, 1985.

Lewis, T., F. Amini, and R. Lannon. *A General Theory of Love.* New York: Random House, 2000.

Linde, P. R. *Of Spirits and Madness: An American Psychiatrist in Africa.* New York: McGraw-Hill, 2002.

Luhrmann, T. M. *Of Two Minds: An Anthropologist Looks at American Psychiatry.* New York: Vintage, 2001.

MacDonald, R. A. *A Country Doctor's Chronicle: Further Tales from the Northwoods.* St. Paul: Minnesota Historical Society, 2004.

Mayhew, M. "Review of Acetaminophen Overdose." *Journal for Nurse Practitioners* 3, no. 3 (2007): 186–88.

McHugh, P. R. *The Mind Has Mountains: Reflections on Society and Psychiatry.* Baltimore: Johns Hopkins University Press, 2006.

McQuistion, H. L. "Challenges for Psychiatry in Serving Homeless People with Psychiatric Disorders." *Psychiatric Services* 54, no. 5 (2003): 669–76.

Monahan, J., et al. "Developing a Clinically Useful Actuarial Tool for Assessing Violence Risk." *British Journal of Psychiatry* 176 (2000): 312–19.

Osorio, R., et al. "Predicting Recidivism after Orthotopic Liver Transplantation for Alcoholic Liver Disease." *Hepatology* (July 1994): 105–10.

Ramchandran, V. S., and S. Blakeslee. *Phantoms in the Brain: Probing the Mysteries of the Human Mind.* New York: Quill/HarperCollins, 1998.

Rasmussen, N. "Making the First Antidepressant: Amphetamine in American Medicine, 1929–1950." *Journal of the History of Medical and Allied Sciences* 61, no. 3 (2006): 288–323.

Rouse, J. D. "Borderline and Other Dramatic Personality Disorders in the Psychiatric Emergency Service." *Psychiatric Annals* 24, no. 11 (1994): 598–602.

Sacks, O. *Vintage Sacks*. New York: Vintage, 2004.

Sadock, B. J., and V. A. Sadock, eds. *Kaplan and Sadock's Comprehensive Textbook of Psychiatry*. 8th ed. Philadelphia: Lippincott Williams & Wilkins, 2005.

———, eds. *Kaplan and Sadock's Synopsis of Psychiatry*. 9th ed. Philadelphia: Lippincott Williams & Wilkins, 2003.

Schumm, J. A., M. Briggs-Phillips, and S. E. Hobfoll. "Cumulative Interpersonal Traumas and Social Support as Risk and Resiliency Factors in Predicting PTSD and Depression among Inner-City Women." *Journal of Traumatic Stress* 19, no. 6 (2006): 825–36.

Scott, K. *SoMa*. New York: Kensington Books, 2007.

Selzer, R. *The Exact Location of the Soul: New and Selected Essays*. New York: Picador USA, 2001.

Shea, S. C. *The Practical Art of Suicide Assessment: A Guide for Mental Health Professionals and Substance Abuse Counselors*. Hoboken, NJ: John Wiley and Sons, 2002.

Shinichiro, H., et al. "2-Nonenal Newly Found in Human Body Odor Tends to Increase with Aging." *Journal of Investigative Dermatology* 116 (2001): 520–24.

Siegel, D. J. *The Developing Mind: How Relationships and the Brain Interact to Shape Who We Are*. New York: Guilford Press, 1999.

Simon, R. I. *Bad Men Do What Good Men Dream: A Forensic Psychiatrist Illuminates the Darker Side of Human Behavior*. Washington, DC: American Psychiatric Press, 1996.

Simon, R. I., and D. W. Shuman. *Clinical Manual of Psychiatry and Law*. Washington, DC: American Psychiatric Press, 2007.

Surman, O. "Psychiatric Aspects of Liver Transplantation." *Psychosomatics* 35, no. 3 (1994): 297–307.

Talesnick, I. Audiotaped interview by author, November 2006, San Jose, CA.

Taylor, A. D. "By My Own Hand." *Bellevue Literary Review* 6, no. 2 (Fall 2006): 117–21.

Thompson, H. S. *Fear and Loathing in Las Vegas: A Savage Journey to the Heart of the American Dream*. New York: Vintage, 1971.

Tolle, E. *The New Earth*. New York: Penguin, 2007.

Towle, C. *Common Human Needs*. 1945. Reprint, Silver Spring, MD: National Association of Social Workers, 1987.

Tyrer, P. "Acute General Psychiatry: Too Hot in the Kitchen?" *Psychiatric Bulletin* 26, no. 5 (2002): 3–4.

Viscott, D. S. *The Making of a Psychiatrist*. Greenwich, CT: Fawcett Publications, 1973.

Volkow, N. "Drug Abuse and Mental Illness: Progress in Understanding Comorbidity." *American Journal of Psychiatry* 158 (2001): 1181–83.

Williams, W. C. *The Autobiography of William Carlos Williams*. New York: New Directions, 1951.

Williams, W. C., and R. Coles. *The Doctor Stories: Compiled by Robert Coles*. 1932. Reprint, New York: New Directions, 1984.

Wolfe, T. *The Electric Kool-Aid Acid Test*. New York: Farrar, Straus and Giroux, 1968.

Text: 11/15 Granjon
Display: Granjon, Bank Gothic
Compositor: International Typesetting and Composition
Printer and Binder: Sheridan Books, Inc.